What's Eating You?

A STEP-BY-STEP GUIDE TO FINALLY
TAKE CONTROL OF YOUR EMOTIONAL EATING

KELLY N. BREWSTER, WHNP

WESTBOW
PRESS®
A DIVISION OF THOMAS NELSON
& ZONDERVAN

Copyright © 2022 Kelly N. Brewster, WHNP.

All rights reserved. No part of this book may be used or reproduced by any means, graphic, electronic, or mechanical, including photocopying, recording, taping or by any information storage retrieval system without the written permission of the author except in the case of brief quotations embodied in critical articles and reviews.

This book is a work of non-fiction. Unless otherwise noted, the author and the publisher make no explicit guarantees as to the accuracy of the information contained in this book and in some cases, names of people and places have been altered to protect their privacy.

WestBow Press books may be ordered through booksellers or by contacting:

WestBow Press
A Division of Thomas Nelson & Zondervan
1663 Liberty Drive
Bloomington, IN 47403
www.westbowpress.com
844-714-3454

Because of the dynamic nature of the Internet, any web addresses or links contained in this book may have changed since publication and may no longer be valid. The views expressed in this work are solely those of the author and do not necessarily reflect the views of the publisher, and the publisher hereby disclaims any responsibility for them.

Any people depicted in stock imagery provided by Getty Images are models, and such images are being used for illustrative purposes only. Certain stock imagery © Getty Images.

Edited by Pam Eddings

Cover design by Bunkerboy Productions

ISBN: 978-1-6642-7052-7 (sc)
ISBN: 978-1-6642-7053-4 (hc)
ISBN: 978-1-6642-7051-0 (e)

Library of Congress Control Number: 2022911820

Print information available on the last page.

WestBow Press rev. date: 09/08/2022

Contents

Acknowledgements vii
Introduction xi

Part I. Finding the Emotional Monster in the Room

Chapter 1   One Bite at a Time! Finding the Tipping Point 1
Chapter 2   The Emotional Monster's Bio 12
Chapter 3   P.R.E.P. The Next Step 21

Part II. The P.R.E.P. Steps

Chapter 4   Perception: Music to My Ears! 29
Chapter 5   Rationalization: Busy is My Middle Name 44
Chapter 6   Expectation: The Ultimate Shell Game 56
Chapter 7   Preparation: Living in Hurricane Alley 69
Chapter 8   What's The Plan, Stan? The PREP FOR
            IT Program 80
Chapter 9   Slips, Trips, and Pitfalls 101
Chapter 10 Exercise: The "X" Factor 111
Chapter 11 "The Game-changer" Emotional Health
            and Well-being 124

Part III. From Soup to Nuts: PREP FOR IT 6-Week Starter Course

Assembly Required 139
6 Week Start-Up Course Overview 143

COVID, Corona...Tomato, Tumato Afterthoughts 241
References and Background Reading 245

Acknowledgements

I often make the comment (in my best Gru voice), "If I had a few minions, I could rule the world!" However, a huge feat or accomplishment is never done alone, but by the combined efforts and sacrifice of many. "*What's Eating You*" is not any different. Although the idea for the PREP acronym and concept of the book may have been conceptualized in a Condo on the Marina, it took numerous months, the right test subjects, and many headaches and sacrifices to birth this incredible outcome.

First and foremost, I thank God for giving me this amazing opportunity to utilize this precious gift that He has bestowed upon me. James 1:17 (ESV) says, *"Every good thing given and every perfect gift is from above, coming down from the Father of lights, with whom there is no variation or shifting shadow."* I thank Him for His grace and mercies that abound, each and every day. We are all given a precious gift from our Father, don't leave it in the beautifully wrapped box. Moreover, I urge you to wear out every bit of your gift until the wheels fall off!

I thank my sweet family, especially my sister, Tracy Evans, for offering encouragement when needed, an enduring love that has taken us all through many victories and yes, even the most difficult of trials.

To my sweet Pastor, Paul Trentacoste, and our beautiful first lady, Malinda Trentacoste, I am forever grateful for your love, friendship, and unending support. In addition, I thank my Pastor for offering himself up as a willing test subject for our many PREP experiments. I love our "FAM" dearly!

Every author needs an individual who is willing to yield a sharp red sword or in this matter, a gel pen and with precision cut, shuffle and even discard grammatical and spelling errors to create a more refined product. Much love to my dear friend and editorial knight, Dan Gilliland, who spent numerous hours going through the initial transcript, to produce an amazing initial edited version of this book. Many, many thanks to a new friend and the mastermind behind the final product, Pam Eddings. She made this diamond in the rough, shine far brighter!

Writing a book doesn't just happen over the course of a few weekends, at least not for me. It took a few years of persistence and tremendous support from those around me. I couldn't have gotten through this process without my work family (shout out to Anna Delrio and Michelle Pell) who became incredible sounding boards and helped me through the good, bad, and even ugly days in the writing process. I have a tremendous amount of gratitude and respect for Dr. Katherine L. Williams, who saw the potential in a novice Nurse Practitioner, as well as providing an opportunity to get away and relax that would ultimately become the inspiration for this book. I would be remiss not to thank the multitude of female patients I have had the honor to care for in the last 17 years as a Nurse Practitioner. You allowed me to be a part of your weight loss and wellness journeys, which provided a platform for my personal growth and development in this healthcare field.

Although we shouldn't judge a book by its cover, I am so thankful for such a creative and beautiful team that made the cover, just over the top! Many thanks to Sonya Perilloux for her amazing photographic eye and incredible pictures for the cover, and to our gorgeous model, Allison Brooks for bringing the cover to a whole other level. You guys are rock stars! One of the most arduous tasks a writer can have, is finding the perfect title for their book. One that gives the reader immediate access into the mind of the writer and what the book is all about. This part was truly a struggle, but a patient and friend of mine Angelle Lyman, who I also participated in some HIIT (cough, torture, cough) workouts with, hit a homer right out of the park! She came up to me before a class and said, "You know I have a title for your book. I was praying about it and felt like God put it in my heart!" Before I could even get the words out of my mouth, she blurted out "What's Eating You?" My mouth dropped open, and I was in awe. Unbeknownst to her I had been praying that God would send me or give me the perfect title. That my friends, is what an answered prayer looks like! I truly thank you Angelle for being sensitive to the Lord and having something that was dear to me, on your heart as well.

I would like to thank you, our reader, who took a chance on this concept, and I pray that you are able to create an environment of overall wellness and weight loss that will last a lifetime. Lock that emotional monster in his cage, and please, throw away the key!

Last, and by all means not least, my dear husband Bryan. As I sit upstairs working on this acknowledgement, he is selflessly cleaning the hot mess that I created in prepping our meals for the week! I am so thankful for your undying love, unwavering support, and helping me to "rig up" wings for my dreams to take flight. I love you dearly.

Introduction

To The Moon, Alice!

"The Honeymooners" is a classic sitcom from the early 1950s, when television had just been making its big debut. It featured the main character, Ralph Kramden, who always appeared to be perpetually flustered but incredibly optimistic. He is well-known for the iconic phrase, often directed at his wife, "To the moon, Alice, To the Moon!" Obviously, the implication of this statement was extremely derogatory, but it captured a glimpse of what this character was feeling. Ralph was at the brink. Enough was enough. Of course, this was a fictional storyline, meant to amuse but more importantly impart a fraction of truth into the day-to-day lives of so many blue-collar workers of that era. Many, many individuals will have that same "To the moon" moment in their lives when they are dealing with unwanted weight gain or an unhealthy lifestyle.

Now, there are two types of individuals that will pick up this book and read it from cover to cover. There are those who have moments of clarity; they recognize that there is a need in their life and that changes need to be made. Then there are those who will have the ultimate aha moment, finding themselves literally on the brink. The difference between the two comes down to endurance, discipline, and an unwavering tenacity. Which one are you? Where do you find yourself residing today?

If I can impart anything to you through these next several chapters, it would be for you to find your aha moment. Make everything you plan on doing, worth it for the long haul. Fad diets, gimmick supplements, and trendy eating plans tout fast, easy results. However, we know that something that is truly worth having will come at a cost. It will take sacrifice, tapping into resources and the dedication of your time. However, can I tell you, that if you find that aha moment, that moment where it all makes sense and you have the much-needed epiphany, that is where you will find long-term wellness and weight loss that can become the lifestyle that you have envisioned.

The biggest difference between those who have moments of clarity and those who have the aha moment, is simply a strong desire for change that makes them willing to throw away the cakes, cookies, cokes, and whatever else away and never look back. Moments of clarity, yes you may see temporary success but somewhere along the way, life creeps back in, and the emotions of the day become the catapult to derailment. However, those of you having aha moments, welcome aboard! You are embarking on a journey that will allow you to create permanent changes to your overall wellbeing and even impart some permanent weight loss along the way!

PART I

Finding the Emotional Monster in the Room

CHAPTER 1

One Bite at a Time! Finding the Tipping Point

I needed a break. I had been riding the proverbial hamster wheel with its relentless 90-mile-per-hour pace, for what seemed like years. We have all been there: caring for our families, meeting the demands from work, church and other community endeavors, and getting up the next day to do it all over again. In July of 2018, my boss graciously offered me an opportunity to get away for a few days and stay at her condo to unwind and recharge a bit. Without any hesitation, my husband and I packed a few items. We made arrangements for a good friend to manage the farm for a few days and took a short trip to the coast for a bit of restoration and regrouping. The place was incredibly peaceful. Overlooking the marina, it was a quiet nook in the chaos of our lives at the time. If you are anything like me, it takes a little time to shut the engine off and just idle; sometimes even days for me to be able to truly inhale, exhale, and finally relax. After a day and a half, I began to feel the water and the sounds of the marina impart restoration into my life.

We had a great first day. We walked the marina, got a quick bite to eat and did a little fishing in the evening. The next night, as I was preparing to dive into the incredible soaker tub, I noticed a small, inconspicuous scale in the corner of her bathroom, offering a bit of temptation to take a little peek. As I stood there for a moment, I told myself, "Why not? Let's see how I am doing?" So, I hopped onto the scale, wait for it.... wait for it.... wait for it.... What in the world?!? I was devastated, absolutely devastated. This is the heaviest I have been in my entire life, even after having 2 children. How did this happen? How did I get here? It was incredibly overwhelming. I sat at the edge of the tub dumbfounded and at a loss for words (very unusual for me). At that very moment, my "aha" moment came when I realized enough is enough!

I walked out of the bathroom, sat next to my husband in the living room, and just started pouring out my heart (and my guts) for that matter. Now you have to understand, my husband has always been supportive through every high and every low. He has never once made any comments or done anything to make me feel worse. I do an amazing job with that all by myself. However, you should also know my husband has to jump around in the shower to get wet! He can eat whatever he wants, whenever he wants, and weight can't find him in a paper bag! In fact, if he doesn't eat, he loses weight just by breathing. Yes, seeing this makes you want to print out invites to your pity party; just realize this is a normal emotion when you see someone eating a cupcake and still lose weight! To his credit, he just sat there and listened as I went through a monologue of what can only be compared to sheer mayhem about where I was and how I had even gotten there?! He never offered any suggestions. He simply listened, allowing me to start thinking about, when was I most successful with weight management in my life? When had I felt like I had the most control over weight loss and my overall wellness?

How can someone who was physically fit and active her entire life, now walk around 30 pounds heavier, miserable, and desperate? How does this happen? How do you go from ninety-miles-per-hour to a snail's pace in care of your physical body? These are just a few of the questions I pondered that day. These may be the very same questions you ask yourself, over and over again. Honestly, I don't have an absolute answer to any of these questions, but I have some very strong ideas about what it takes to get to that point.

I know what you are thinking, "Kelly, 30 pounds really isn't that bad. Look how tall you are! You really don't look overweight. You just look, well…um, healthy! You are so busy, it's too hard to add one more thing to your life right now!" Seriously, I have heard it all, and I have said it all to myself and anyone who would listen. You don't get to this point overnight. You don't wake up and look in the mirror and say, "What on earth has happened?!" You get here one small bite at a time, and guess what? That is how you will get the weight off: one bite at a time. To some, this change in weight and overall wellness may have seemed very sudden, but it is a slow process that creates a big impact. So many times, I have conversations with my patients about their weight gain. Actually, it is probably one of the most popular topics next to no sex drive, and that really is a topic for a whole other book! Patients come in, either living in the silent despair of where they have landed along this weight-gaining journey, or the polar opposite occurs when they have a full-blown melt-down in my office. Now, you have to understand something. I am a Nurse Practitioner in Women's Health. The majority of what I diagnose and treat is below the border, but over the past 15 years, I have found myself developing programs and teaching plans that have provided assistance to individuals struggling with metabolic conditions leading to chronic obesity. How ironic, huh? I have helped thousands of women successfully address their metabolic issues while secretly dealing with my own internal struggles with emotional eating. Some say that could be hypocritical, but in all fairness, sometimes it is easier to apply the oxygen mask to those around us and fall incredibly short in applying the appropriate measures for our own safety. Can I get an Amen in the house?

You see, what is so "mic-dropping" about these conversations is that we will actually obsess about the THOUGHT of losing weight, changing our lifestyles and eating habits, but we really are not willing to DO much about it when the rubber meets the road. When I am having these conversations with my patients, one of my favorite sayings to use is, "How do you eat an elephant?" (Now you must be careful here because if they think they are significantly overweight; this could put you in hot water in a heartbeat!) Most patients will look at me like I either just woke up or they are trying to figure out what turnip truck I just fell off. Others know exactly where I am going with this. Of course, the answer is…one bite at a time.

For you to truly know what brought me to this place of resolve, the place where enough is enough, and there is no day like the present, I need to take you back in time, way back to the beginning before I had a care in the world, about staying physically fit and healthy. When I was growing up, I literally could eat a dozen chocolate cupcakes before dinner and still eat dinner and not gain an ounce. By no means am I bragging, well maybe just a little, but weight management wasn't even on the radar for me at that time. I was extremely active: always outside, always involved in one competitive sport or another. Life was good! In college, I tried out for the volleyball team; that was my sport of choice throughout junior high and high school. I played for two years at the University of Southwestern Louisiana, now known to most as the University of Louisiana Lafayette. I remember finishing two 3-hour practices a day, driving home and stopping at the 7/11 store to grab Hot Tamales and a Tab. What a combination! Between my first and second year in college, I started really developing an interest in physical fitness and training off season. I actually became obsessed! I would run to the training facility, which was about 2 miles from my house, weight train and then run home. I was very diligent with food choices and counted calories, incorporating Low calorie frozen meals (these were just hitting the market at that time) several times during the week. I was extremely regimented, striving to make the healthiest choice possible for myself. In the off season, I needed to get a job for a bit of spending money. So where did I attempt to get employed first? You guessed it, a gym! I taught aerobics a few times a week, and it gave me access to weights when the training facility was not available. When we checked in with the coach to start our preseason training, she had the athletic trainer take out these plastic pinchers (it was an instrument to measure the fat content on your body) and everyone had to be evaluated. I literally had gotten my body fat percentage down to 15% between my freshman and sophomore years. So much for the freshman 15, huh?

    During college, I met my first husband and had my first child, Reid. I stepped away from the collegiate arena, but this did not stop me from focusing on my health and fitness. I would put the baby to bed at night and work out to videos in my living room. Changing it up, I would bike in the morning before work, and there was really a short stint of roller blading in the morning. That did not go over very well (the shin pain was seriously more than I could bear!). Believe it or not, I was thinner after having my first baby than I was after training for my sophomore year of volleyball. At one point, my mother was concerned that I had cancer, because I would not eat and the baby, who was about six months at the time was as wide as me (Reid's nickname, monster-baby!). I didn't have an eating disorder. I really just wasn't hungry, and when I did eat, well, I was trying to eat healthy, creating new, healthier menus, all while sticking to my southern roots.

Even after a divorce and having two children, my focus remained steadfast on health and fitness. I would workout at least 4 times a week, started playing competitive tennis for my cardio workout, and continued to consume healthy, balanced meals. With just a bit of an obsessive nature, I would play tennis 3-4 times a week in the evenings after work. Even playing a bit of racquetball; you name it, and I was playing it. Thinking back, my kids were really gym babies. I often toted them with me to the gym after school and work. Meanwhile, I always kept a pulse on my eating habits and tried my best to either count calories or increase my workouts, and focus on increasing my consumption of all the right foods.

We are getting there. I promise! So, fast forward to 35 years old, new marriage, still extremely active and as always, eating healthy. I was very methodical with my eating. It was, without a doubt, a function. In fact, it was border-line mundane and boring in many cases. I ate the same scrambled eggs or peanut butter toast on 11 grain bread for breakfast, and then grilled chicken salad for lunch, day in and day out. Although my fitness regimen had started to slow down just a bit, I was still extremely diligent with my eating habits. I always had at least one component of healthy living in check. Now I will say this; I love to cook! In fact, I love to cook almost as much as eating; well, almost. At this time in my life, I started experimenting with recipes, creating new menus, preparing different types of ethnic foods, and venturing outside of my Cajun comfort zone. Of course, when you cook the food, you must eat it! However, even at this point, I was still maintaining my healthy weight. Why? I was still strict with breakfast and lunch and would not prepare these meals routinely. They were highlights to the week.

Everything changed on July 6, 2006. You see, up to this point. I had experienced some trying events. Some things had the opportunity to curtail me, but I had never experienced a traumatic event in my life. I had read about them and heard about them. I just had not experienced them. I received a call from my mom on that Thursday evening to inform me that my young brother, Ronnie, was struck by lightning and was in critical condition. She asked that I come to the hospital immediately. You have to understand for the purpose of this book, I had never understood what made individuals eat emotionally. I had never understood what made people turn to food for comfort. Yes, I liked chocolate and candy, hello?! They are my staple at times, but I didn't use them for emotional comfort. I just didn't understand the draw toward food as a comfort until now.

You see, as a Nurse Practitioner, I knew what critical condition meant; I knew what the chances of recovery were when you are struck in the head by lightning. I believed my brother could be miraculously healed, so I was not really prepared for his death. On Friday morning, at 7:20 am, the critical care physicians at the hospital requested a conference with the family and started the conversation with, "Ronnie has had a lot of damage to his heart and suffered from a heart attack this morning." I was, still waiting for, "but he was resuscitated." Instead, the physician says, "we were unable to save him."

What? You mean my 30-year-old little brother was gone? I was devastated, truly devastated. We got through the wake and funeral as many would... numb... dazed... and still living in disbelief.

My life as an emotional eater began at that moment. I didn't run straight for the vending machine or hit the nearest fast-food restaurant. It happened very slowly and very inconspicuously. I would go into the media room just to eat a box of Hot Tamales or Whoppers. I stopped cooking and preparing meals and became very reactive in my food decisions. I attended to my grief by eating when I wanted, what I wanted, and how much I wanted. You see, I couldn't bring my brother back, but I could control what I ate, and it became my comfort. Through the course of a year, I went from a comfortable size 8, to living in a size 12. This didn't happen overnight. It was really a very slow trickle effect, lulling me with a bit of false reassurance that all was still well. Still, the bill comes due for us all, and eventually the comfort eating caught up with me. I would look into the mirror and become even more grieved that I was out of control, and what would I do? You got it. I would go back to what made me feel comforted, safe, and better. Even if it was for just a moment. The old adage that says *"a moment on your lips; forever on your hips"* was likely written by someone who had dealt with the same emotional beast I had let out of the cage. What happens in this case, is that you initiate what is called a positive feedback system. In other words, you create a vicious cycle that resembles a boulder rolling off a cliff, heading to the bottom at the speed of light. We will talk about this feedback system in the next chapter of the book.

Here is where it gets even more interesting. You see, once you feed a particular emotion, (in my case, it was grief; for you it could be stress, fatigue, anger, or even depression.) the body in essence attempts to provide for you when the extreme emotion is initiated. Your body tries to anticipate what you need before you attempt to seek out the remedy.

You may say, "Ok Kelly, I'm confused."

Alright, think of it like this. Originally, I ate because I was grieved, bereaving the loss of my brother, but what started as a response to grief eventually became a response to any extreme emotion. For example, when you are extremely happy, you want to celebrate with what? Food! Having a very stressful day? Nothing a little dessert can't fix, right? Maybe you are really angry about something, nothing like a venti Frappuccino to show them! Starting to get the picture? The body attempts (with good intentions) to alleviate the intense emotion with the one thing that has worked in the past. It anticipates the need for comfort food, and it creates a craving or strong desire to eat certain foods. It would be awesome if it would drive you to a green apple or quinoa, but no, it sends you to what it knows you like best: cookies, candy, pasta, or bread.

Now, I won't say that I didn't try and snap out of this and attempt to use an eating plan or fad diets to get back to a healthy weight. I would lose 10, maybe even 15 pounds and then just the smallest extreme emotion would knock me off of the plan and back to square one. Coincidently, I was dipping into my 40's, making any attempt of eating healthy and exercising far more laborious than it had been in the past. It started taking longer to see progress and as a result, became even more frustrating. Know this; eating plans, like any plans that we have, usually have a beginning and you guessed it, an end. This occurs because you either get tired of following the diet plan, or something derails you off of the plan. (Things like a birthday, holiday, or special occasion; any event that allows you to rationalize eating outside of what is healthy for you and "splurge.") One special moment becomes one special weekend. This then becomes one uncontrollable week that can inevitably throw the plan out of the window and let the emotional beast out of the cage. Again. Better yet, try living in South Louisiana, a place that has holidays associated with food. Wait! What I mean is food associated with holidays, family events, and any celebration that will inevitably come along. We have food for graduations from kindergarten, christenings, and funerals. Oh, you made an A on your final? Let's go celebrate! You get where I am going with this. These are just barriers to getting back on the road to success.

I did use an eating plan that is associated with network marketing and had some success with it. I lost 22 pounds! Off to the races! That was short-lived, however. When my mother became sick and within months was placed in hospice, the emotional monster started banging on the bars of the cage to come out and play. The 22 pounds I had lost found me rather quickly and brought a few friends along. I didn't realize what was happening at the time. I just knew that I was in a funk, and I was struggling to find a way out.

I kept the weight on until a friend told me about an eating plan focused on whole foods and the concept behind this plan. The day after Christmas in 2016, I left all abandon behind and moved forward with the plan. The next day while watching some football with my husband, I looked at him and said, "You need to throw that white chocolate cake away. I am going downstairs to put my face in it!"

He looked at me for just a moment with a bit of a grin and then realized that I was absolutely serious. He quickly trotted downstairs to get rid of the temptation. That first week was brutal. I was as mean as a snake because the sugars were being purged out of my system. The emotional beast was angry that he was being forced back into the cage. By day 7, I was on top of the world. I had lost 4 pounds and by the end of 30 days, I had lost 12 pounds and continued to lose a pound a week after that. I was extremely strict with the eating plan during the week and would allow myself a cheat day on the weekend.

STOP!! This is where the train derails. I didn't have a traumatic event at this point, but every time I had an extreme emotion, my body would send me looking for comfort food. This, by the way, is NOT on my eating plan, and I started to slowly succumb to fate.

Sitting in the beautiful condo, overlooking the Marina, I reflected back on my life, to my successes and failures with weight. I realized my true successes came when I was adequately prepared. When I strategically planned my meals and snacks for those special events and occasions. When I took the time to get in the kitchen for just a few hours a week to prep my food, schedule my meals and what I would eat, I removed the ability to react negatively to an extreme emotion. As my husband and I talked, my mind started racing and literally the PREP FOR IT program was born that day, in that living room, overlooking the marina. We talked about the concept of the acronym, what each of the letters mean and how this could not only get me back on the right track, but also potentially help others who have the very same issues I have dealt with throughout my life.

Figuring out what got you here, what has created the "YOU" at this moment, is really the first step in the right direction for permanent weight management and living the healthiest lifestyle you can. I was always the one who would skip the first 3-4 chapters of the book to get to the meat (excuse the pun) of the issue. I strongly urge you not to move through the book quickly to get to the details and start the program. Go through all of the acronyms and what they mean in your life. Sit down and truly reflect on what got you to this point. This could be one of the hardest lessons that you will learn in this book because it is finally confronting the emotional monster that pushed you to this point. Seriously, take some time and think about what got you to where you are right now. What worked, and what were your biggest obstacles? Then work through each of the acronyms so that you can set yourself up for the best long-term success. I had to remember that the emotional monster that creates cravings and causes us to dive into a negative spiral of carb frenzy has to be trained to stay in the cage. You do this by preparing every step of the way.

Before moving into the next chapter, I strongly encourage you, yes pressure you to sit down and write out your testimony. Find out what exactly tipped you off. When did the emotional monster start whispering in your ear or knocking on your door and offering you a few ding dongs and sodas to make you "feel better"? You truly need to be able to identify the tipping point in order to start moving forward through the P.R.E.P. steps to regain a fitter, healthier you!

Your Tipping Point

Understanding the past can create a better view into the future. This often requires a trip down memory lane. The purpose of taking your personal testimony and writing it out on paper, is to see, in black and white, what triggered your emotional eating. What actually catalyzed that moment in your life that opened the door to these emotional ups and downs, and finding a starting point to establish your goals for success.

Attempting to forego this exercise is truly doing yourself a great disservice. Without knowing the moment or event that got you to your present state of mind and yes, body, the potential for success with this program is unfortunately, limited. It may help you to meet some initial goals. Even help you to see some weight loss success. However, to have a game-changing moment in your life, you need to pull back the curtain and address the Oz in the room! This can be a brutal exercise to work through, but so are burpees, and we do them when the coach tells us to do the reps so…

Drop and give me that testimony! (Recommendations: review the course of your life, significant events such as a death of a loved one, a stressful job or situation, financial hardships, divorce, etc. We all have something that catalyzed our emotional eating, it's just a matter of digging it up.)

_____

_____

_____

_____

_____

_____

_____

_____

_____

_____

CHAPTER 2

The Emotional Monster's Bio

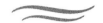

I am not going to lie; just putting my testimony into words can make the emotional monster throw a temper tantrum and start whining in his cage. But, identifying that he is there? Well, that is the first step in ensuring that you are on the road to a really successful, healthy lifestyle. See, I think this is really what we need to understand. The emotion that triggered binge eating, bad choices, and excessive carb intake will always be just one extreme issue away. It may be a bad day at work, difficulties in a relationship, or not having a really balanced life. The list is endless. It's how you control your response to the emotion that becomes your biggest weapon and will allow you to maintain long-term success.

So, let's go back to where PREP began. When I sat in the living room of the condo and started venting, I mean talking to my husband about where I was, how I got there, etc., etc., etc., I realized that the time in my life where I experienced the most success was when I was adequately preparing my meals. I mean, it really hit me like a ton of bricks or maybe sponge cakes. Use your imagination! It is such a liberating moment when you realize the wizard behind the curtain controlling your food cravings and prompting your bad choices is just a puny little thing looking to take advantage of you in your vulnerable situation. I realized (get your highlighter for this one) that when I provided an environment to proactively plan, I found myself making less of the reactive choices that eventually lead to bad habits. So, planning looks something like this:

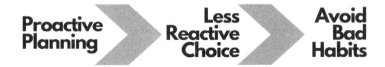

Let's use this in context, shall we? You have decided your New Year's Resolution is to finally, I mean finally, start shedding the holiday weight, the summer weight, and last year's holiday weight. (By the way, never, and I mean never, decide to do this on New Year's Day. The day you decide you want to do it, that is the first day you should start. Now, where were we?) Okay, you browse through many different diet options, and there are plenty out there to choose from. You find one that seems to fit your needs. Maybe it's the next best seller on the market and you go to work. You do great the first week. Yep! People at work may have secretly had a pool going to see how long you would go, but you, my friend, are holding strong 4 days into the new "plan." It's Friday and you wake up a tad later than usual. You did not have a chance to pack your usual snacks to ease you through the work day and figured, it's just Friday. I got this. I can wing it!

STOP! First mistake, we never, and I mean never want to wing it if at all possible. When we are unable to complete the first component of this equation, we essentially prevent the rest of the equation from coming into play. So, if we would look at the same formula in a slightly different way, when we are making reactive choices in lieu of the proactive ones, the equation starts looking something like this:

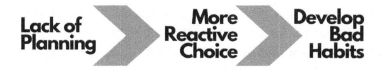

Back to the story: So, it's Friday. Your co-workers are talking secretly in the back of the office. You walk up and ask what is going on? They blurt out that the boss is wanting to meet with the staff in an hour, and the project that was supposed to be turned in on Monday has to be presented in an hour! Imagine this scenario in your head with me; panic ensues and the extreme emotion called stress knocks on the back of your brain saying, "Mind if I stay awhile?"

You scurry back to your desk, sit down to start feverishly putting together your best proposal, not realizing that you are working through your mid-day snack. Of course, since stress is the emotion in charge, you appease him with a good old bag, I mean, a few Hershey kisses lying in wait at the bottom of your desk. The proposal now complete, you present it to your Boss who raves about your finished product, and then the whole office heads out for a bit of a Friday lunch celebration. You have now taken the emotional monster from a fit of pure stress to a peak of great excitement in less than half a day. You are now not just hungry, but you have triggered the emotional monster numerous times through the course of the day, giving Him Carte Blanche with food temptations and cravings. With your boss, who is treating everyone in tow, you sit down with the group. You know what thought runs through your head, don't you? You deserve to splurge today. You worked hard, and it calls for a celebration. Eat whatever you want, it's ALL GOOD!" "He gave me the biggest compliment today on my proposal. You know a raise can't be far behind! Bring out the good stuff!"

Now your EM (emotional monster) is encouraging you to react and make a choice you would otherwise not make. Co-workers exchange glances (as well as money) when you decide on the bacon cheeseburger on the brioche bun with a side of fries. Of course, it hits the spot, and why yes, I would love to see the dessert menu!

BOOM! You are in the Reactive Zone, and here is where you need to be extremely careful. Failing to recognize these emotional reactions and letting your guard down, little by little, opens a window for those small, bad habits to become much larger contenders and then, let's face it, game changers.

How can that be, Kelly? I simply splurged for one meal. How is that a game changer?

Well, I am so glad you asked! You see, when you did not proactively plan, you set in motion a trigger response that we will break down into medical terms in just a few minutes. When you did not ensure that the meal you were prepared to eat was nutritionally balanced, fit within your daily caloric intake, and was just a function within the day, you woke up the ghrelin (hunger hormone) release in the body. This essentially has the potential to fuel additional carb cravings within a few hours of eating this particular meal. In addition, now that you have LISTENED to that voice taunting and tempting you and responded to it, you have created an opportunity for him to wreak havoc when your next emotional swing occurs, and so the story unfolds.

As you leave the lunch meeting, you head home to get your weekend started early with just a little guilt about your food choices, only now you walk into the house and realize that the new puppy you just adopted has gotten into the trash. Garbage is now spewed throughout the kitchen, living room, bathroom, yep, it's the whole house! It's a hot mess, and it doesn't really smell any better. You are angry, frustrated, and discouraged as you begin the daunting task of cleaning up the house. After you finish picking up the last of the chaos, you remember that you have a half-eaten pint of ice-cream (that didn't get thrown out when you started the new eating plan) still sitting in the freezer. That's when you hear it! *It's okay; really it's okay. We have the perfect solution for you. It has been a very stressful day, one for the record books, and that little bit of ice cream is the perfect way to make you feel better.*

Guess what? In that moment, the ice cream does make you feel better because you have become an emotional eater, and anytime you experience an extreme emotion, your body will make every attempt to rectify the situation and bring you back to center. To make you feel better, (emotionally anyway). Sometimes the response to the emotion occurs solely because you may not be able to control the changes around you, but you can control what you eat and what may improve your mood. This tells the monster that you will feel better when allowed to be comforted by foods and things that make you feel better, even if you know deep down it is not really what is best for you. This response creates a cycle that is extremely hard to break.

I told you that we would break this down medically so you can get a visual, right? In medicine, we call this a positive feedback system or loop. Also known as an exacerbation loop, it is defined as a process that exacerbates the effects of a small disturbance. By no means do we see it as a positive concept, but the way it is directed through the body is through this feedback system. So, it looks something like this.

You have an extreme emotion, and you respond by comfort eating (this is typically a carbohydrate heavy meal and often lacks the necessary protein to create the balance or nutritional value that is needed for weight loss and improved health). In order for your body to process this appropriately, it will need to break that carbohydrate down into a usable fuel, and this requires your insulin level to dramatically spike upward. Once this occurs, you will process the meal that you consumed and as a result, the insulin will drop just as suddenly. This will cause you to feel like you are still hungry, grumpy, and maybe even a bit tired. It will inevitably give you a desire to head back to the pantry for a quick remedy which, in turn, notifies the body to produce more insulin, causing you to go around the mulberry bush yet again. These sluggish, sleepy, and sedated feelings you are experiencing are like the bat symbol in the Batman movies. It is signaling the body to remediate the issue with whatever means possible to get the body back to a homeostatic (balanced) state. How will it do this? You guessed it! It will elicit an insatiable craving (increase the ghrelin) for comfort foods and yet more carbohydrates.

Now this diagram looks very technical, but it really provides a great understanding of the way that both positive and negative loops occur in the body.

Feedback Loops

Positive Feedback Loop
Recognizes a change and amplifies it.

Negative Feedback Loop
Recognizes a change and brings it back to normal

To fully understand what is going on, let's use something that most people can definitely find relatable. You log into your bank account the day before payday to just check in and make sure all of the transactions and checks have cleared. You remember you just gave a $30 check to a fellow employee for a church fundraiser before you left work yesterday. When you look at your balance, it shows a current balance of $25 dollars. The next thing that happens is a RESPONSE to what you just saw: PANIC! Your heart will start racing, your mind will kick into overdrive and immediately attempt to rectify this situation as fast as possible. Since you did not put overdraft protection in place, you immediately transfer $100 dollars from your savings into the checking account. Your heart rate has now decreased, your stomach acids have calmed down, and life is good again. This, my friends, is a negative feedback loop. In most cases, when you eat healthy, the same thing is occurring. You eat a healthy meal, and it stimulates the insulin production; the food is then broken down into a sugar that is used by the body. As the sugar levels in the body come back down, the insulin release "valve" is shut off, allowing the sugars to return to normal ranges. This is the one time that negative can be a positive thing!

Now a positive feedback loop is quite different. It is a cycle that basically feeds into itself. A great example of this feedback loop would be a reward system. Even if you don't have children, we were all there at one time and, believe it or not, we were part of an operative called the star reward system. You're not sure what I am talking about? Ok, let me break this down. It is third grade and you are a bit of a Chatty-Kathy, and your teacher just started a star reward system. If you paid attention in class and participated, you got a star. If you didn't talk in class, you got a star. If you did your homework for the next day? You guessed it! You got a star! If at the end of what felt like a long week, you had at least 8 stars, then you would be able to go to the special flame-throwing event all the kids were talking about. So, what did you do? You faced forward, finished your homework, and got a star. That motivated you to raise your hand in class because you wanted to get more stars. You were not going to let anything distract you from that ultimate goal.... going to the event! This is a positive feedback system. In your world right now, when you feed the extreme emotion with a reactive choice, it reinforces that behavior, and when you experience the next extreme issue or event, then the system is already in place to create the reaction. Hence, the positive feedback system.

Understanding that once we have catalyzed this feedback system in the body, any extreme emotion has the potential to elicit a similar response. There is an array of emotions that can trigger similar responses: anger, stress, frustration, elation, and many other emotions that will prompt the body to find the solution that brings it back to "center." We have provided some examples of different emotions and what you may find when the body responds in this feedback system to the emotion you may be experiencing.

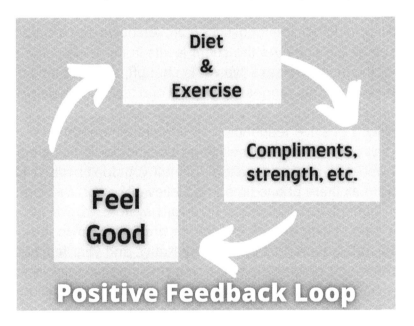

Don't get me wrong; this could be a very healthy loop if it started with diet and exercise, reinforced with confidence and strength, which then made you feel great and encouraged you to diet and exercise further. We have all experienced this particular feedback system: mentally geared up to make a change in our life, starting to see a change in our energy, strength and even in our weight. In order to keep this particular feedback system "positive," it is imperative that you implement strategies to prevent derailment of these positive changes.

Now back to the story. As you are finishing the last bit of the ice cream, (Yes, you decided, why get a bowl? I will simply eat it from the carton. Please, you know you have done this before!) This is where you can find yourself on a slippery slope without any means to get you back to safety. As you sit slumped over on the sofa, empty ice cream carton in hand with the all too familiar sugar daze, you feel guilty, discouraged, and frustrated. Again, all of these feelings can lead to extreme emotional swings that could catalyze the next ice cream run. This is how a positive feedback system works. It will continue to feed itself until someone, (that would be you) decides enough is enough and breaks the cycle and creates the necessary change.

What is imperative in this situation is not only trying to change the feedback system itself and make better overall choices, but also to get the epiphany that food is not an occasion or activity. It is a function. Wait! What? Yes, food should be just a function. It provides the fuel and energy that our bodies need to get things done through the course of the day. Food goes into the body, and, well you know the other part of the story. Over time, we have attached emotion to food. It has become the center of most, if not all, occasions and even part of our entertainment. Food does have a place in social settings. In fact, the Bible talks on more than one occasion about people fellowshipping together with the breaking of bread. However, one should also take note that gluttony is a sin. You see, the difference between the two scenarios is that fellowshipping and getting together with loved ones for a very important event may occur once or twice a month, or even a few times in a year. However, it's not when your 8-year-old has successfully completed a book report on his/her own, or you were able to leave an hour earlier from work, so let's grab some sushi. Seeing food as a function and not an occasion will give you a tremendous advantage in taking on the monster with proactive planning and prepping your way to a healthier, leaner you!

So, how did I get here? I mean, I wasn't always like this, Kelly!?!

In most cases, people haven't always been this way. What?! I wasn't always this way! Over time, when you allow yourself to emotionally eat with either the possible lack of physical activity, a change in your eating plan, or an increase in your caloric intake, it can create a climate for the emotional monster to roam freely in your life when making everyday food choices. Basically, any cycle, whether positive or negative, had to start somewhere. Something catalyzes the reoccurring events. Finding the event or moment when the cycle began is imperative to breaking the positive loop that inevitably creates a downward spiral. That is where the testimony we covered in the last chapter is so important. You need to know where all of this started so it can provide an avenue for your best long-term success plan.

In order to provide a mechanism for combating these core issues, I developed an acronym that walks you through a process that should put a leash on your emotional monster. In the next chapter, we are going to provide an overview for the PREP FOR IT system, briefly discuss the acronym and how it works, and then provide more in-depth discussion about each of the PREP FOR IT components. I know you are ready to get there. However, in order to provide you with the best opportunity for success, it is absolutely imperative that you understand how to identify the triggers by utilizing the best tools from the plan, and providing the best opportunity to attack.

CHAPTER 3
P.R.E.P. The Next Step

My Pastor, who is a dear friend of mine, once gave a sermon titled, *"Desperate Times Call for Drastic Measures,"* and I will say with all sincerity, I have applied this teaching to my life on more than one occasion. Find your point of desperation in your life, and find the motivation you need to implement some drastic measures to improve the situation. (For me, it was the moment I stepped on that scale.) We can get lulled into thinking that everything is okay as long as we are bringing everything back to center after emotional swings and binge eating go out for a night on the town. But truth be told, we are only being conditioned to ACCEPT the extreme emotional shifts and responses that ensue. I love the analogy of the boiling frog. Now, I realize for the pet lovers out there, and I am one of them, this seems morbid. However, if you take this in context, it makes so much sense. When you place a frog in tepid water, they are happy, content, basking in all of their glory. Little by little, you slowly warm up the water and the frog, well the frog adapts. Given enough time you can bring the water to a boiling point, and the frog never jumps out. The frog has become conditioned to the environment that surrounds him as well as the constant exposure to harmful triggers that will lead to his ultimate demise. He may be in a desperate time, but he has created an environment that is not prompting him to take the drastic measures he needs to save his own skin.

We are no different than this frog. Instead of us soaking in a Jacuzzi, we fall into this slow fade of reactive decisions, eating those cookies in the break room, going through the drive through out of sheer convenience, and celebrating with a nice meal because our child just finished their science project with two days to spare! All of these poor decisions lead to bad habits, and then one day we wake up, wearing nothing but elastic waist bands and leaving the boutique with a new cute purse or earrings because that is the only thing that fit comfortably in the dressing room!

Remember what I said in chapter one, you have to get to a point of resolve; you have to get to the moment that you plop down on the sofa and say to yourself and anyone else around you who wants to listen; "Enough is enough!" It's time to implement the drastic measures that it will take so that you can finally, and I mean finally send the emotional monster packing.

I mentioned in the first chapter that I reached my "AHA" moment at my bosses' condo after the scale sent me into a tailspin that was going nowhere real and I mean, real fast! As I sat there talking with my husband about the successes and failures, the one thing I was always drawn back to was, when I was sufficiently prepared, I had less mishaps. Really this happens with anything in life: studying for a test, going to an interview, or finishing a project at work on time. Poor planning catalyzes a reactionary mechanism in us that may lead to the most unpredictable results we will experience.

Think about it like this for a second. Let's use the example of getting ready for a corporate event that you are organizing. You have 8 weeks to prepare for this big event, but you find yourself chasing the inevitable rabbit and doing other things instead of chipping away at the to-do list. When you realize that you are behind the eight ball folks, it's kind of too late. You now must be reactive, and you are running around in a frenzy the week of the event to pull it off like it had been planned for months. You may snap at a fellow co-worker for no reason, become a tad more negative during that week, and instead of being employee of the month for a job well done, well, you may wind up in the bosses' office, discussing your need for an attitude adjustment. A good bit of this, probably all of it, could have been avoided simply by taking a few minutes each week to eat the elephant, one bite at a time. Preparing to undergo a change in how you approach food and the choices that we make when it comes to eating healthy, is really not any different. We can glean a lot from our resilient rodent friend, the squirrel as he is feverishly planning for the winter, scooping up as many nuts as he can before the first wisp of winter starts coming in. He doesn't pack all of this in his little den 2-3 days before he needs them. He is planning months ahead of time, collecting a little each day to ensure he has everything he needs for the long, cold days ahead.

Eating healthy and creating successful opportunities for weight loss is contingent on creating an atmosphere for planning and not reacting. Sitting down a few days before the next week and establishing your menu, creating the grocery list and then collecting all of the ingredients to make the next week uneventful at least from a nutritional perspective is essential. When my husband and I sat there and talked that morning, I realized it's not just about the preparation of the food; there are a lot of other factors that play significant roles in making this successful. Hence, the creation of PREP FOR IT.

PREP is an acronym that stands for perception, rationalization, expectation, and preparation. It provides a mechanism to create a platform for your best success. Oftentimes most people will do a little bit of research before starting an eating plan, and then they pretty much run to the deep end of the pool and dive off before learning how to swim. But knowing what your perception is about your weight gain, your eating habits, and even what those close to you see and observe, is vital in creating an amazing foundation for success. Rationalization, the next step of the program, provides you an opportunity to shore up the weak areas of your life and understand how you respond to certain triggers. Most of us are experts at rationalization; in fact, if there was a career in this, many of us would be living large on the products of our endeavors.

The third step is Expectation; what do you expect from yourself, the program, and others. This is a hard one because you did not get where you are right now overnight, and you will not get back to where you were overnight either. I always ask my patients this question: "If I am driving from Louisiana to Florida and I decide to turn around in Mississippi, where am I? I am in

Mississippi! Just because you decide that today is the day you are finally going to drop those sixty-five pounds hanging around way too long, doesn't mean that you will wake up after a week of prepping and jump into those skinny jeans! This is a process; it takes time to create the necessary momentum and long-term success that you want to see.

The last step is the meat; excuse the pun of the process. It is where all of the brass tacks are handed out and where you will live through this process. Preparation is necessary to avoid the pitfalls, the reactions, and the creation of bad habits. Yes, this is where the proverbial rubber will meet the road.

My husband and I worked on a self-owned company for over 5 years, called Healthcare in A Nutshell, a women's healthcare site that provided videos on various women's topics that were taught in terms you could understand. We took his music studio that we built and turned it into a filming studio, green screen, and all, and got to work. Videos provided a way to ensure that all of the information we wanted to convey was comprehensive, and it allowed us to teach in a way that would allow our audience to have fun learning the information and completely understand it. As we sat there in this spontaneous brain-storming session, which by the way, I often do, we realized that eventually, educational videos would be an incredible way to teach others about the P.R.E.P. FOR IT course and how to implement it into their lives.

Yes, the brain child was born here, but it took months of actual planning and prepping, finding out what worked well and then what was more trouble than it was worth. I needed to work on developing and refining the best recipes for success and making sure that they would allow you to be able to achieve the goal of improved health, wellness, and yes, weight loss. But the recipes couldn't just be good; I wanted them to be great. I wanted the participants to feel like they were not missing a thing; in fact, I wanted the recipes to be so good that others around you in the breakroom at work became, well yes, a little jealous. You don't stay committed to something long-term if it's just mediocre or okay; you stick with it when it can WOW you, and that was the mission.

Before putting the program on paper, I needed to find some willing subjects, I mean, participants in my experiment who were at the same point of desperation that I was. Enter, my Pastor. Now you have to understand that my Pastor and his wife are our best friends. We love them dearly, we trust them wholeheartedly, and are submitted to their guidance in our lives. We really are truly blessed by them. But when it comes to healthcare, the roles are a bit reversed. He is very open to constructive feedback when it comes to weight management and wellness, and I found him at the corner of desperation and frustration in relation to his health and weight. He is this incredibly warm and loving Italian man who would tell you one of his favorite hobbies is food. Food for him also had a lot of emotional ties to it. La Familia, right? He admitted that food was an emotional outlet, and it had been a struggle essentially all of his life. Newsflash! If you emotionally eat, you will always have to deal with the emotional monster that was initially let out of the cage; this is a lifestyle change, folks, a career, not a season in life.

This is when you know that you are a kindred spirit because his eyes light up much like mine do when we start talking about food, preparing it, eating it, what restaurants are the best, the list could go on and on. He was on the cusp of his 50th birthday, and he wanted to get back into a healthy state of mind and body before his birthday in 3 months. This meant losing at least 25-30 pounds quickly!

He was at the point of resolve, and I needed a willing subject, so we talked about trying out the prepping, I would cook the meals for both of us, and we would follow the program together and see how it would go. He did fabulous! Of course, the first week was a bit challenging, I think he may have asked me about snacks several times…a day. So, we portioned his meals in the prepping containers, and at the beginning of each week, I would drop his meals off to him. Seriously, he was like a big kid; he couldn't wait to see what was on the menu for the week so he could decide what he would try first! He was not only able to lose the weight, but also realized that the way he had approached food all his life had led him to emotional eating; now he began to see it as a function and not as an event. We needed to change that, and change my friends, doesn't come overnight. Remember, this is a process and for both of us, it was a change in lifestyle that we needed to stick with for the long haul. The funny thing about this is that during this 6-week process, when I prepped for the week, I also included my husband's portions because frankly, there was no way that I would be cooking meals two different ways! So, he was also along for the ride, and he even lost weight! Remember, he is the one that has to jump around in the shower to get wet, however skinny doesn't always equate to healthy, so it helped him from a wellness standpoint as well.

We both reached our weight goals; in fact, even after we finished the 6 weeks of prepping for him, he was so motivated that they implemented those strategies for prepping and weight loss on an ongoing basis. Did we have bumps in the road? Sure! We are human and will have moments in time, and occasions in which our options are limited, but realizing that the emotional monster is there and that we need to always keep him confined to the cage; why, that is half of the battle.

In the next few chapters, we will start breaking down each of the acronyms for P.R.E.P. FOR IT and really delve into the components of each step, what it means in your life, and how to devise a plan that will catapult you into wellness and weight loss success. There is no time like the present, so let's get to work!

PART II
The P.R.E.P. Steps

CHAPTER 4

Perception: Music to My Ears!

It was a blistering cold morning in January 2007, and a young man was playing his violin at the metro station in Washington, D.C. He proceeded to play 6 Bach pieces over the course of an hour. While the music flowed with precision from the skilled musician's hand into the frigid air, almost 2,000 people would pass through that station, many heading to work for the day. A middle-aged man noticed the young man playing and slowed his pace for just a few seconds only to hurry along to meet his schedule. A young man leaned against the wall to listen to him, only to look at his watch and then started walking off again. A 3-year-old boy abruptly stopped in front of the musician, after the young man had been playing for about ten minutes, only to be tugged along by his mother to get to the sitter's apartment. Even though the child was persistent to stop and take in the beautiful melody, the mother was frustrated and pushed even harder to prompt the child to move along. After 45 minutes, and thousands crossing the musician's path, only six people stopped to even listen for just a short while. Many individuals would monetarily contribute to the hat, and when it was all said and done, the young man had collected a grand total of $32. Joshua quietly finished the musical pieces, placed his instrument in its case, and slowly walked away. In the silence no one applauded, no recognition was given to the young man. The young man in the train station that day was Joshua Bell, one of the greatest musicians and violinists in the world. He was playing the most intricate musical piece that was ever composed, on an instrument that was valued at $3.5 million. Two days prior to this experiment, Joshua Bell played at a theater in Boston to a crowd that would garner approximately $100 a seat to a theatre filled to capacity.

This was a social experiment that was organized by the Washington Post and was later published in the post as "A Violinist in the Metro," with the purpose of evaluating people's perception and the context of their priorities. Each passerby had a quick choice to make as they heard the eloquent sounds flow from the tips of the incredibly talented musician. Do I stop and listen, or do I hurry on with my day? Is this a thing of beauty? Or is this just another musician trying to make a living with the bit of God-given talent they possess? The violinist had a preconceived perception about how the experiment would turn out and so did a music instructor who was interviewed prior to the experiment. Even the Washington Post noted their thoughts about the experiment prior to that cold January day. Joshua was inconspicuous, in a pair of faded jeans and an old long sleeve T-shirt. To those around him, passing by, he was just another aspiring musician, trying to make ends meet. To Joshua, he was an accomplished musician possibly attempting to revel in a bit of anonymity, forgoing the formalities of a scheduled concerto. Each person that passed him by, formulated a perception of what they were experiencing and to them, their perception was absolutely accurate!

The first part of the PREP FOR IT acronym starts with how you see yourself, your personal perception. The proverbial reflection we see when looking into the mirror. It is how we truly perceive ourselves, and how we think that others see us as well. Perception is an impression, a way of understanding your surroundings or situations that you may be going through or dealing with at the time. There is a saying I tell the staff I have had the privilege of managing for the past eight years when referring to customer service and unmet needs.

"A patient's perception is reality."

Despite what they may have done or not done, if a person has preconceived perceptions about a situation, it is difficult to present alternate possibilities or concepts to them.

Truly the best example of this is what happens after the fender-bender occurs. Not that this has ever happened to me; perception, right? So, an accident occurs, the police are notified, and arrive within a few minutes of the occurrence. In your mind, you have recounted the event through your eyes and unbeknownst to you, the other driver is developing a similar recollection from their point of view. When the officer arrives and asks for a description of how the accident occurred, you give an extremely detailed version of the event, going all out with a remarkable rendition of charades, using exaggerated hand motions and facial expressions as you tell your perception of the event, through your eyes. Then in awe, you sit silenced by the reminiscent portrayal of the event by the other driver, who by the way, has sick skills in articulation and rendition of the event, leaving you stunned and confused.

How could someone see things so differently? How could she not see that she was slow to indicate her turn or quick enough to avoid the collision? Inevitably, the officer will hear two very different perceptions of what transpired. This is not to say that one person is lying and the other may not be. It really is two different views from two different people from two different places and somewhere in the middle is reality.

Just as the social experiment done in the L'Enfant Metro in Washington D.C., everyone has the opportunity to formulate their version of what they experience in their day-to-day lives as well as how they choose to react to these established perceptions. This is one of the main reasons why we live in such a divided country, at this time. By no means is this stated to initiate robust dialogue on our individual political beliefs, but the way we FEEL about something determines how we will ultimately perceive an issue and hence, develop a form of reality that in our eyes becomes absolutely correct. The older woman who slipped a dollar into Joshua's hat, as she hurried along, may have perceived this young man as someone who needed a little helping hand, but she may have felt burdened or a tad guilty that she couldn't lend a hand in the rush of her day. So, the contribution may have accommodated some needed relief from a bit of maternal guilt. The 3-year-old was enamored by the music and the flow of the bow across the strings, engrossed in the musical notes; however, the mother's perception was that this was an unnecessary distraction that impeded her ability to get to her next destination on time.

The issues that can arise when perception becomes our reality, especially with wellness and emotional eating can contribute to that vicious cycle that we talked about in Chapter two. We often do not realize how much our perception about our health, what we are eating, or even how we look really affects the reality of where our mail is delivered every day. I would like to call this the *cupcake phenomenon.* We eat a cupcake for a special occasion, and we wake up the next day feeling fine, dress fits well, I don't see a change in the mirror, so all is good. The next day you may have a celebratory dinner of some sort, and of course, you indulge and eat all of the courses including a peek at the dessert menu. We wake up, yet again fitting in our clothes just fine; nothing looks different from our view into the mirror, and off to work we go.

Our perception? All is well; none of these activities have had a negative impact on my progress. Then, there is a birthday lunch at work today, and they have your favorite cake for the birthday girl; so what do you do? Well, you can live on the wild side because let's face it, you look great; you can still zip up that skirt or pair of jeans without sucking in, (well, maybe just a little bit) and your reality that you are living in is now being affected by your perception that everything is A-Okay! Sure, you will have a café-frappe whatever with extra whip cream and caramel, well, you don't mind if you do. We talked about the slow fade a few chapters ago, but honestly it starts with one choice. One choice that can send you down the proverbial rabbit hole.

Now I am not implying that you cannot ever have an opportunity to indulge, but when you do, you must understand that you need to see it for what it is. The reality is, you may be making a reactive choice or a bad choice that could affect you in some way even if you do not PERCIEVE a change in your wellness or weight at that time. So, if you are mindful of the choice and how it will affect you, then it in turn will prevent you from being blindsided by the change in your wellness or appearance in a month or two, if you are able to stop the freight train before it leaves the station. I am not implying that your ability to celebrate with a meal or a dessert is forever erased from your future; what I am saying is that you need to look at it for what it is and respond to it appropriately. Change your perception about how you look at that activity, and it can very well change future reactive decisions. This will not be easy. Societal tendencies, especially in the South, have attached significant emotional ties to the food we eat, why we are eating it, what we are eating, and yes, even how much we are eating. As we discussed previously, fellowshipping, with friends, over a fine celebratory meal is good for the soul when selective; but when it becomes the norm, it can quickly create a perception or expectation that every meal should be emotionally driven, feeding into the vicious cycle. When you are faced with making a decision on whether you are going to eat the food that is an unhealthy choice, or outside of your proactive meal plan, ask yourself, "Will this help or hinder my goal?" Sometimes just a time-out to actually think about the decision is enough to counter what you would have initially decided.

So, Kelly this is great and all, but how is identifying my perception of myself really going to help me obtain the wellness and weight loss that I truly desire?

Great question, and the perfect place for change to begin. There are several questions I would like you to really think about, maybe even jot down some things that resonate in your mind when you read these questions so we can make sure that your perception of your wellness and weight management is closely aligned to the reality that you live in day in and day out.

How Do I See Myself?

One of the first questions I would like you to ask yourself is, "How do I see myself? When you look in the mirror, what do you see? As humans, we typically have a tendency to hone in and focus on the negative parts of our appearance and don't give ourselves credit where credit is due. When you look at the overall shape of your body, realistically look at the primary shape that your body resembles. Some are pear shaped, apple shaped, egg shaped and triangularly shaped. Most are under the assumption (perception) when you go on a weight loss journey to shed the unwanted weight and to slim down to the fighting weight you would like to be, that you will lose primarily in the spot of greatest trouble.

In reality, when we lose weight, we lose it throughout the body and will typically show the first signs of weight loss in the areas where we have a tendency to have more water or fluid retention. On the many weight loss journeys that I traveled, I know that I have a tendency to initially lose weight in my face. Inevitably someone will come up and ask me, "Have you lost some weight, your face looks thinner?" As I am sure you can only imagine, the first week of your healthy eating journey can start out on the bumpier side. You may be a tad feistier, as you are working over the emotional monster with better meal choices and calorie restriction, regaining the much-needed control.

What do I want to say to the question? "Why yes, I have. As a matter of fact, I am losing weight because all of my turtle necks were getting too tight!" Really?!? Of course, I don't always respond in that matter (sometimes, possibly) The reality of weight loss is that it may take some time to see some notable changes; just keep in mind what the ultimate long-term goal may be and stay the course. Something else to ponder, relative to our appearance is to ask yourself, "Do my clothes fit comfortably?" If not, where is the issue?

I caution you about the "yoga pants" syndrome. This particular incident occurs when an individual will slowly start to infuse their normal wardrobe with clothing items that have spandex or elastic as the main textile. Their "perception" is that the clothing that is conforming to their shape, that has incredible give, is flattering and comfortable, thereby they begin to incorporate several similar garments into their existing wardrobe. As a result, many individuals that struggle with weight gain may have 10 different pairs of yoga pants that become their go-to for any occasion. Worse, many of these individuals will sadly succumb to the "yoga pants" syndrome and allow the comfort of the clothing to create a false sense of security with their wellness and weight management, becoming completely overwhelmed with their sudden but necessary reliance on spandex products. I work in a medical office seeing patients throughout the day and wear scrubs when I am in the clinic, along with my lab coat. If you have ever worn scrubs, you know that there is a false sense of security and comfort in relation to weight gain. Scrubs are meant to fit loose and continue to fit loose, until they don't, and by that time, you are in a heap of trouble!

Grasping the reality of "wear" you are at this time, allows you to begin the much-needed transition into realizing where you actually "fit" into your wellness and weight loss plan. There are several additional questions I would like you to think about when it comes to perception and how to obtain a better sense of reality as we make our way through the PREP FOR IT process.

Do I consume good nutritious calories, or am I eating empty calories?

Truly doing a bit of introspection here and rating your overall food consumption, can help to pay high dividends in developing the foundation for long-term success. During the many weight management counseling sessions that I have had with patients, I asked them what type of foods they find themselves eating. The funny thing when asking this question is the responses I often hear. Some patients start off with, "I usually eat very healthy." Others offer the following responses: "I just eat what is available when I get home." "Well, I am a picky eater, you know." "It's so hard to eat healthy, but I try!"

I have seriously, heard it all! Many of these responses are vague, reveal the nature of the patient's perception about their food intake and how misled they find themselves, and quite frankly, a few of the responses appear to be oxymorons. You are either eating healthy, or you're not. You are either making good food choices, or you're not. You are either trying, or you are not. This can be a game changer for you. When you pull the "be real" card out of the deck and finally play it, you realize who has been misled all along. Be true to you! Ask yourself the hard, rhetorical questions, and give yourself honest answers. When you do, it allows you to make the changes to the eating plan that are necessary for your success.

Do I limit my food options based on past experience?

"I didn't like Brussel sprouts before, so I know that I won't like that recipe, Kelly!"

How often have you found yourself steering away from foods that you have consumed in the past, simply because the food experience was less than satisfying? You may be missing out on opportunities to experience new tastes and experiences based on limited exposure in the past. How were they prepared when you had then last? Did they have organic bacon or pork back tossed in them? Were they caramelized on the edges? Okay, I may be drooling a bit at this time, but you get my point? Clean the slate on past perceptions so it allows you to open up the door to new options and opportunities.

I love my mother more than anything and miss her dearly. She was a good cook, but our veggie dishes lived on the corner of boring and mundane avenue. I remember eating the same three or four vegetable combinations prepared the same way each and every time. Shaking things up and providing variety to your food choices can actually open up a whole new world to the food repertoire that you have at your fingertips. Additionally, we need to keep in mind, that as we age and mature, our palettes have a tendency to do the same, and what we would have preferred to avoid in the past, may inevitably become your next favorite meal!

Do I emotionally eat?

Now this is a big one, because it can become the most significant catalyst for weight gain and unhealthy eating habits quicker than anything other issue. Do you envision yourself "to be or not to be" an emotional eater? Is your current self-perception the epitome of an individual who takes the bull by the horns and moves on with life, no strings attached? While observations from those around you tend to lean toward a scenario where you head to the vending machine as soon as something at work appears to go awry. Knowing whether you are an emotional eater is truly the biggest part of finally containing the emotional monster for good. What happens when you are faced with a significant, sometimes life-altering situation? Think about this for a moment. Did you reactively eat? What type of response did you actually have both during the event itself, and then when the smoke cleared and the dust finally settled?

Ask yourself, "If I am an emotional eater, what is the main emotional trigger for me at this time? When you begin to take the steps to identify this, it becomes easier to put mechanisms in place to prevent the emotional triggers that catalyze the reactive eating choices. Remember, once you have started to emotionally eat, your tendency is to comfort eat for ANY extreme emotion however, finding the initial trigger and dealing with it can truly create the platform for long term success.

Do I exercise?

There are many questions to ponder when analyzing how you may perceive your wellness and weight loss in relation to your exercise regimen. "Do I exercise on a regular basis? Am I as physically active as I need to be?" If so, what is my perception of what I am doing at the moment? I have patients who come in to the office just for their well visit, and the main question that will inevitably come up is, "What can I do about this weight gain that I have?"

I ask 3 simple questions that, honestly, we should be asking ourselves, perhaps weekly.

1. Are you exercising?
2. Are you eating the right foods and avoiding the wrong things? (This includes alcohol here!)
3. Are you eating the right number of calories?

The answers may vary, but one thing is certain. When it comes to answering these questions, the person who lives with the response, day in and day out, is you. Be honest with yourself; it means the difference between long-term success, and hitting the ice cream aisle again within a week or two of your new eating plans. Many individuals perceive that the functions they execute at work can be classified as exercise.

"I move around a lot at work Kelly. I am always on the go and rarely sit down." "I lift heavy boxes throughout the day," or (this is a good one!) "I sweat a lot at my job!"

Really?! If our physical fitness was predicated simply on whether we get a good perspiration going, then every menopausal woman out there would be a size 2, living the high life! We will not belittle this point since we have an entire chapter dedicated to this topic, but rather use this time to become candid with yourself in relation to your present level of physical fitness and what is your perception of your physical fitness level based on what is actually occurring at this time.

Where is kitchen on the map?

Another question that I would like you to ponder is, "How comfortable am I in the kitchen with cooking and preparing food?" You may think that you are not much of a cook or chef, but given the opportunity to follow a little guidance and sound recipes, you my friend, may tap into an undiscovered talent or hobby that you may actually find enjoyable. Being open to experimenting with different seasonings, ingredients, and even utensils will give you more confidence in your abilities and will have a tremendous impact on sticking with a sound eating plan and enjoying the journey along the way! Please realize, it doesn't take an expert skill-set to conjure up a week's worth of healthy, balanced meals that can set the platform for proactive planning and long-term success.

Now that you have evaluated your perception of where you are and what you have been doing, let's put pen to paper. Let's dive into the reality of the situation and where we are actually living.

You have probably already started to read your own mail and get a more realistic picture of what your wellness and weight loss picture looks like, but there are a few more things we need to cover in laying a great foundation for success. I like to affectionately title this part of perception, The Reality TV phenomenon. Many have been enthralled by this new type of entertainment that gives the viewer the impression that the reality TV program we are tuned into is what is actually happening to these individuals that are being filmed, almost as a documentary of sorts. But in reality, most of what the viewer is being enamored with is simply scenarios concocted by producers and writers to gain ratings in the TV world. Yes, the individuals portrayed in these series may be real, but the essence of the actual program has been pre-planned and written to draw you into the experience. I want to discourage you from getting the reality TV mindset about where you are in this weight loss and wellness journey. I want you to get a full documented, factual recount of where you are living and how it has affected you. It is imperative to take the rose-colored glasses off to see what is actually happening, not what you or others may perceive to be going on in this journey.

To get the foundation laid for true success, you will need to put actions to your plan. I am always jotting down notes or drawings for any projects that I want to make a reality. I even have a drawing pad that has many sketches for the dreams of the future (I believe that my husband would love nothing more than to "misplace" the notebook at times, so the projects slow down just a tad!) So, grab a notebook and let's get to work. First, you need to start logging in your daily calories for at least a week, to get an idea of where we need to address the biggest offenders first. If you are not a pencil and paper person, I get it. There are a lot of smart phone apps that do the majority of the work for you even to the point that you scan your item in, and it documents calories, carbs and such. Journaling food intake is one of the best ways to get an idea of just how far off of reality you really are living.

The next thing you need to do is going to hurt, but I promise in the end, you will love me for it. Take a picture of yourself. Yes, a candid full frontal shot of yourself, maybe in workout clothes or something that will let you see your true shape. Next, use the body shapes provided in our supplemental workbook and find your shape. The reality of how you are shaped will help you to understand that when the changes do occur in your body, you will reduce the size and maybe some of the curves, but it may be difficult to completely change the overall shape. You were uniquely made for a purpose, so even if you don't have that hour glass type shape, let's make you the best pear-shape that you can be, right!

One of the most crucial parts of documenting this journey is what got you here in the first place. You wrote your testimony in chapter one, which is absolutely essential to change your mind-set toward food, but you need to really document how you feel in your day-to-day lives; what is causing the most harm to your wellness and weight loss? Is it frustration at work? Is it the stress of getting the kids to activities and functions after work? Is it the recent loss of a loved one or a divorce? Yes, these are significant things that will have a direct effect on your potential emotional eating, but what about the smaller bouts of emotional swings? Document how you are feeling and whether any of these feelings triggered a need to comfort eat. What was your initial, gut response to the pendulum swing of emotions in the course of a day? This particular exercise will truly enlighten you to what essential requirements are needed by you to lay a sound foundation for success. Remember, one of the biggest keys to long term success here is remembering to make eating a function, not just an occasion or activity. Trying to remove as much emotion from eating as you can, permits you to detach from the food and see it for what it really is, just fuel to continue with your day!

Finally, what encourages me the most?

For so many on this journey, the scale can be your enemy or your friend, depending on the day and time. I discourage my patients from taking daily weights because honestly, our weight can vary from day to day, or hour to hour for that matter. Since our weight is a daily variable based on several factors, if we are not careful, we will start chasing numbers instead of wellness, and it can sabotage your success just as quickly as our friends Mac and Cheese! Are you someone who is positively motivated when you start to see your clothes fitting differently? If so, make sure you are allowing yourself time before trying those smaller clothes on because this can be counter-productive as well. Be realistic. Try the turtle necks on first!

Do you get more positively motivated by compliments from others? This one can be a bit of a catch-22. Do not ask a question of someone if you are fearful of the answer; you may be looking for words of affirmation and instead, you get a big dose of reality or even worse, pessimism that will do nothing to drive positive momentum on your wellness and weight loss journey. Choose your questions and the timing of those questions wisely. Be your own cheerleader here! As you start on this PREP FOR IT journey, note all of the positives that you are getting from the PROCESS. This is just as important as the outcome. How do you feel physically, mentally, and even emotionally through the process? Noting what makes your days' successes and some opportunities, allows you to continue to build on your foundation for long-term success.

World's worst chef or Emerald's worse fear?

One of the last questions I would like you to ponder as we move through the PREP FOR IT process, is "What is my perception of my ability to cook and prep in the kitchen? What is my skill-set when it comes to chopping, dicing and Juliann carrots? That last one was just for fun, but seriously our perception of what we are capable of accomplishing may be very different from what we can actually do once we decide to get in there and operate more than just the microwave! In chapter one, I mentioned that I am from South Louisiana, and we love everything and I mean everything about food, which is what makes this process even more challenging, but interestingly, I was not taught like others how to actually cook. I did not find myself in the kitchen watching my mother whisk up the next Better Homes and Gardens meal during the week. So, how did I begin to master some of the skills in the kitchen to be able to prep efficiently and still have a meal that makes me want to drive home rather than go through the drive thru? It took practice my friends! It took getting in there and learning what the different utensils were for and what worked and yes, what didn't work before Stella got her groove on! You may have heard this saying, "if you say you can, or you can't, you will," or maybe this one, "where there is a will, there is a way!" You, my friend, have taken a tremendous step forward toward your long-term wellness and weight loss goal. So, whether you are the student who is already familiar with the functions of the stove or how to puree a cauliflower, or on the flip-side, you may not be sure what the difference between dicing and mincing an onion are, you both can obtain the same level of success with the PREP FOR IT process because you have decided to make a change in your life, and that really is the hardest part of this whole process. That doesn't mean that preparing and prepping your food will be super-easy, or that you will come out of the kitchen when you are done like you haven't worked at all.

No. You may feel pretty tired after getting your game-on and putting the weekly plan in place. But here is what I do know. When you walk out of the kitchen each week, you will feel empowered, you will feel that you can accomplish this mission for the next week, and much like our furry friends that gather nuts for the winter, you will feel prepared! Preparation prevents the emotional rollercoaster from wreaking havoc on you in the upcoming week! To quote one of my favorite people, well more like characters, "You can do it" (said in my most authentic Cajun voice)!

Now that we have had the opportunity to gain a better perspective of where our reality lies, we need to move into the next part of this process and that is Rationalization. In this next chapter we are going to confront this sneaking emotional monster that would like nothing more than to see you stay exactly where you are and avoid any positive changes that could lead to better health. However, before scurrying onto the next step in the process, take a few minutes and go through the activities in the supplemental workbook of this chapter and work through the questions on perception, and how close to reality are you truly living in regard to emotional eating and overall wellness in your life.

CHAPTER 5

Rationalization: Busy is My Middle Name

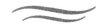

There is an Aesop's Tale called the Fox and the Grapes. The fox walks up to a vineyard and sees these scrumptious, plump grapes hanging from the vine, and all he can think about is how deliciously sweet those grapes will be when he can eat them. He makes several unsuccessful attempts as he slips on his saliva to get to the grapes. He jumps first. Then he takes a running start, leaps, only to fall short again. He does this several times and finally looks at the grapes in disgust. Sitting under the low hanging grapes he says, "What a fool I am. Here I am wearing myself out to get a bunch of sour grapes that are not worth all of this effort!" He proceeds to pout as he walks off, scornful and pessimistic. Hence the term, sour grapes! The moral to glean from this fable, is there are many who pretend to despise and belittle that which is beyond their reach. I would like to go a step further and state that we will make excuses and rationalize what we THINK we are unable to obtain or may have failed to gain up to this point. It's a protective mechanism that we use to provide an avenue for us to justify the final outcome. The fox gave up. He left feeling defeated and discouraged, as he justified his failure by making the object of his affections appear inedible. Many times, we attempt to try different eating plans, exercise programs, and even weight loss medications, only to rationalize the ineffectiveness or the lack of scientific evidence to substantiate the success of the program or product because we failed to obtain the end result.

Rationalization, the second component of the acronym, PREP FOR IT, addresses the ever-present need to justify why we may have eaten that particular meal, or why we are unable to implement some form of exercise into our health regimen. Many, most, well for that matter, probably all of us have even rationalized why we are at an all-time high when we hop off of the scale stunned and in disbelief. Why, even I have made fat jokes about myself! Humor is just one method that we will incorporate into our artillery of Rationalization to ensure that we are justified in staying in a complacent state of mind. Getting through this particular part of the PREP FOR IT process may be one of the most crucial components of achieving long-term wellness and weight loss. The ever-present inner voice wants you to think that staying on the sofa and relaxing is a luxury that you deserve because of how hard you may have worked. This is a dangerous liaison that can lead to a lifetime of unhappiness and perpetual food-binging. Rationalization is quite the modern-day phenomenon. It allows complacency, mediocrity, and settling for "just okay" in life. We will meet numerous people throughout our lives who settle for less and make excuses why they didn't get that promotion, why they couldn't pass the test, or why they didn't marry the love of their life. In fact, making excuses and giving up is a much easier road to travel than the bumpy road of "making it happen." Rationalization can make the present reality an easier pill to swallow even if it's not an ideal situation. You see, this is where the emotional monster is all too happy to assist you in justifying every cupcake, scoop of ice cream, and every single bite of chips and salsa you feel that you need or, deserve. Identifying where you fall in this particular step, how rationalization truly affects and sabotages your long-term goals and wellness plan, is imperative to being able to create a platform to strive for the harder things in life. (Weight loss, wellness, or even a life-long aspiration). When you are faced with the decision to eat something you shouldn't or make a healthy food choice, you have at that moment two ways that you can respond. You can ask yourself, "Is this the best decision that I can make?" or "What could I do differently next time?" Or, you can pull out the big artillery called rationalization, and blurt out, "Say hello to my little friend," and go to town making up justifications for your blatant disregard for the proactive plans that you set in place. If you are unable to relate to what I am stating in regard to Rationalization, here are a few examples of what someone rationalizing may say to the ear willing to listen:

"It wasn't my fault. 'WE' didn't have anything else to eat in the house!"

"If I go to gym today, I will get all sweaty, and I want to be able to meet up with my friends later."

"I felt bad that she was the only one eating the donuts at the office, you know?"

"I am so busy right now with kids, work, and after-school activities, I just don't have the time right now.

"Well, since I ate that ice cream sundae with extra syrup and whipped cream, I will just restart my eating plan next Monday" (said after eating the meal on Tuesday?!).

"What?!?" I didn't bring my lunch with me today, so sure I will go to the Chinese buffet with you. Sure! Why not!"

"Everyone is raving about that new eating plan out there, but I hear there is a lot of cooking involved and you know, I don't even know how to boil water!?!"

There is literally an inexhaustible list of excuses that if utilized, will certainly lead you onto a path of impending health and wellness doom. Let's face it, rationalization is simply one's ability to provide an excuse that seems plausible in your own mind and when repeated enough, becomes completely sensible and appropriate. Rationalizing is just that. It is making excuses for bad choices, allowing you to avoid the hard work to get to the long-term goal. It can either squash your motivation to get started on the road to long term wellness, or sabotage you just a few short miles from the terminal. Excuses make it even more difficult to get back on the road of creating an environment for success and can lead you down a path of "it will do." What does that mean, Kelly? Well, no one wants to be someone's, "He/She will do," right? You want to be the one they have dreamed about all of their lives, and you finally showed up on their doorstep. "It will do" creates an atmosphere of mediocrity that will prevent you from ever reaching the goal that you initially intended and could very well create an internal mechanism that will allow you to rationalize excuses for more than just healthy living, but for anything else in your life. These types of choices can often breed further failure and can even result in depression and long-term health problems. Again, it starts with just one. Just one excuse, just one reason why this bad choice is okay. One opportunity to rationalize why I am not able to complete the workout today. Same slippery slope, just a different mountain!

It is about time to address the elephant in the room and ask him to leave! We all really want to be the best version of ourselves and everything seems good on paper or in our minds, but what separates those who do and those who don't is.... well, excuses! True commitment to long-term goals can be hard to achieve, but what we do on a daily basis can make all the difference in reaching that pinnacle of wellness. Taking responsibility starts within. It is in these moments that you have a sparring match in your mind on which story you will ultimately tell yourself when you may have failed or felt overwhelmed, and what voice you decide you WANT to hear. If you are truly overweight or out of shape, do you tell yourself that all of the women in our family are shaped like this, or do you tell yourself I am still working on finding the solution that works best for me? Or maybe, all of the men in our family are large and in charge! Seriously think about this for a minute and begin to ask yourself the hard questions.

Rationalization is not just about the big, life-changing choices. In many ways it's about all of the small, day-to-day choices that we make and what version we choose to tell ourselves. You know, I see this, ALL of the time in our medical practice. As my patients articulate their newest reasons for not reaching their weight loss goals, I sit back and listen, then think to myself, "Do they realize that what they are telling me does not change anything in my life, but it may be life-changing to them?" We may place blame on several different things in our lives as to why we are not able to achieve long term wellness and weight loss.

To work through this step in the PREP FOR IT process, take a few moments to think about what are the possible excuses or areas that you may place blame for the choices you have been making? I have listed some possible reasons, but really take the time to think about some of the reasons you have been on the side-lines instead of making big plays in the game!

Common reasons may be:

Work Demands	Relationships
School requirements	Limited Resources
Household duties	Monetary Limitations
Time with Spouse	Other _____
After school activities for children	

Ask yourself, "Do I rationalize my food choices and if so, how could I respond differently to avoid making the wrong daily choices?" Do I prepare my food ahead of time, but when the rubber meets the road, find myself still making bad choices once I take a break for lunch at work?

As I sit here writing this chapter, I am not immune from self-evaluation when it comes to assessing my desire to rationalize bad choices. If you have ever had to pick up the pieces after the emotional monsters wreak havoc in your life, then you are susceptible to rationalize or justify your actions, both good and yes, bad. Many times, I have found myself evaluating previous choices I have made during precarious or stressful situations, and wondering if I made all of the right choices.

I am presently at my aunt's kitchen table working on this book, as she is sitting in the recliner battling stage IV lung cancer. Since our available family resource pool consists of a whopping 2 family members, my sister and myself, it would really be so stinking easy to make excuses as to why eating ice cream tonight would be great. It would appear to be practical to say, "It's ok to eat fast food since we have been busy doing other things in regard to her healthcare. In fact, we could justify the need to avoid exercising during this incredibly stressful time by simply saying, "It has just been too hectic to be able to make time for the gym." All of these formal explanations are really just excuses disguised in pretty, easy-to-accept packaging, topped off with a big, beautiful ribbon!

Life will inevitably happen. You will encounter bad days and even worse days. Getting a handle on how you deal with the day-to-day choices will certainly payoff high dividends in your wellness and weight loss goals. Yes, your ability to call out the issues in your life can have a profound impact on how you respond to these unfortunate and possibly traumatic events which have the potential to let the emotional monster have his day in the sun.

Removing rationalization from the equation takes effort. It requires you to stare at the man or woman in the mirror and say "NO MORE!" It means that you have to consciously make an effort to speak the right things into your life and avoid what seems easy to say on the surface. I like reading non-fiction, a little bit of fiction, (let's face it, I love to read!), but I love reading self-help books on everything from spiritual wellness, physical and dietary health, and even financial wellness. What truly frustrates me when I read many of these books, is that they go on and on about how the book is going to change your life, and the strategies in the book will forever change the trajectory of your future, but when I get through to the end, I wind up asking myself "Where's the beef? Where is the meat to this? Where are the strategies to truly make the changes that I need?"

Part of working through the PREP FOR IT acronym is to make sure that when you get through the process, you are energized and enthusiastic about the changes you will be able to make, but more than this, I want you to feel equipped to be able to implement strategies into your life successfully!

In an article written by Malia Frey, *How to Overcome 5 Psychological Blocks to Weight Loss*, identifying the roadblock is the first step in the process to create a better environment. What excuse are you using that will cause the quickest and greatest derailment to your weight-loss goals and start working on alternative measures? Malia identifies a few barriers to overcoming weight gain, and we will take these factors and break them down a little further.

All or None Thinking

You see this all of the time: at work, home, even with friends. Inevitably, there is someone in your life, maybe even you, who, when they decide to indulge in a hobby or activity, they just jump off the high diving board into the deep end of the pool and go all out with a new trendy eating plan or exercise program. They take on the activity full force for a period of time, and then, all of a sudden, you got it.... crickets. They have either moved on to the next best thing, or explained why the present system is not "all that and a bag of chips." We may all possess a bit of this mindset, but there are those around us who take this to the extreme.

A dear friend of mine, who is very vibrant, a total type A personality, will get completely enamored about a new activity, and when she jumps in, there are typically no parachutes involved. Once she wanted to start playing tennis, a novice, but she bought the most expensive tennis racket, designer tennis bag, super-cute outfits and started adjusting her schedule a bit to accommodate the demands of the new activity. As quickly as she jumped into this new hobby, she stopped going and to my recollection, she has not been back. Frankly, we are all guilty of this at one time or another. My husband and I have this running joke. You see we are known as the "DIYers," "Construction Junkies," and "Project Pushovers." Remember that I can elicit cringe-worthy responses from my husband simply by saying, "Babe, I have an idea." So, when we decide to build a vegetable garden and greenhouse, or construct our own chicken coop, we develop incredibly detailed and elaborate plans, and typically what was envisioned does become a 95% reality.

What? That sounds a bit peculiar, Kelly! How can you have a dream or idea that becomes 95% reality?

Well, much to my husband's dismay, we get through most of the projects and when it comes to the few finishing touches, well, we get a bit disenchanted and move on to the next potential venture before we ever COMPLETELY finish the current mission. To our friends, this is extremely comical and the subject of many, many jokes. For us, it is a never-ending frustration.

So how do you combat this? What measure can be helpful in making sure you stay away from the Dr. Jekyll and Mr. Hyde mentality? How can you prevent the "all or none mentality" in regard to your wellness and weight loss journey? Small changes really create the biggest impact.

Start by making a few of the PREP FOR IT meals each week and remove sodas from your eating plan. Once you do that, in a few weeks, start making the main dishes for the week and add 15 minutes of walking after dinner into your regimen, while continuing to eliminate sodas. Eventually, start focusing on your proactive snack planning. You are turning an ever so small snowball into a massive sphere of success. Basically, those subtle changes really create the environment for the best long-term success.

In James Clear's best-selling book, *Atomic Habits*, he paints a picture of what a 1% difference in parts of our lives can do for the overall betterment of the person. He starts by using the example of the British cycling team that was forever changed in 2003. A new energetic coach by the name of Dave Brailsford was hired to change the landscape of British cycling, and that he did. For over a century, the professional cyclist in Great Britain had suffered from patchiness in the sport. From the Olympics to the Tour de France, no one had brought home a title. Mediocrity was the name of the cycling team's game. Dave was hired to change the course of Great Britain's team and was given carte blanche to do whatever he deemed fit to make changes. What made Dave different? It was his relentless commitment to a strategy called "the aggregation to marginal gains" which essentially looked at making the smallest of improvements in each and every part of the sport to create a momentum of positive outcomes. They changed everything from bike seats, to the fabric worn by outdoor riders, even minute things like what pillow and mattress would allow the bikers to get the best recovery and sleep. Again, the purpose was to create small changes in all parts of the cyclists' lives to create an increased overall advantage, and you guessed it! Not only did they see the small, marginal improvements in performance, but they also produced amazing overall results. Just 5 years after making many small, marginal changes, the British Cycling team dominated the road and won 60 percent of the gold medals in the 2008 Olympic Games. Four years later, they set 9 Olympic and 7 world records and won the Tour de France within the same year.

So, you may not be a professional cycler, but the small 1% changes you make in all areas of your life will pay off in big dividends down the line. Again, as we mentioned earlier, stop drinking sodas in the evening, then eventually all together, and you have made a small change that will pay greatly on the back end. Making these small changes in your eating, preparation, exercise, and overall wellness will not only create positive momentum to reach the long-term goals, but also create an atmosphere to reduce the need for rationalization by setting tangible, realistic short-term goals. If you are doing well on your eating regimen and decide to have dessert at dinner on Friday, identify it for what it is and avoid attempting to rationalize the reason for the activity. Simply make provisions moving forward to minimize revisiting this issue in the future.

Chicken or the Egg

The common idiom, "Which came first, the chicken or the egg?" refers to a situation where it is nearly impossible to decide which of the two things caused the other one to occur. Negative self-image, how we see ourselves, can create just another vicious cycle. How many times have you caught yourself looking into the mirror and immediately fixate on the areas of your body that are not the most profoundly positive features? We have a tendency to gravitate to the more problematic areas of our physique. How did that make you feel? Some people will listen to the negative comments that they subconsciously speak into their lives, and it causes them to have a desire to emotionally eat or engage in a number of potentially negative activities.

Ultimately, it may increase the desire to comfort eat and then they are back in front of the mirror to take another one for the team! Again, it goes back to the fox and the grapes, if you do not identify what is discouraging you, then it creates a barrier to your success. I would like to recommend here that you do not weigh yourself for at least 4-6 weeks. I know this may sound absurd, but if you want to truly see results, the scale is the last place you may want to look for evidence of positive changes in the beginning of this journey. Instead of looking into the mirror to self-analyze, try putting sticky notes on the mirror to motivate you to achieve the wellness and weight-loss goals you would like to achieve. I have a great motivational exercise that I will employ when I have a patient who has a high BMI (Body Mass Index). I will ask them what is their initial weight goal, and then we will calculate how much they will need to lose to reach that goal. I then ask them to buy the same number of marbles and place them in one jar and have an empty jar next to the full one (if their initial goal is to lose 25 pounds, then 25 marbles are placed into the first jar). I instruct them to move one marble, for every pound that they lose, over to the empty jar. If they lose 3 pounds, 3 marbles. You get where this is going. You may not feel the difference of 10 pounds when you initially try to lose weight, but when you see 10 marbles moved over into the empty jar, it drives the momentum to keep the positive motivation going. Creating positive changes along the way, will reduce the need to use rationalizations.

Calm Instead of the Storm

If stress is the emotional trigger for you, then proactive planning will become your biggest ally when the stressors occur, and, let's face it, they will occur. Finding an alternative activity or preparing healthy snacks (keeping then conveniently tucked into different places like your desk at work, your purse or gym bag) can help you make better choices when the trigger occurs. Identify areas of your life where stress seems to occur more frequently and make some changes to those areas to reduce the chance for the stressor to actually occur, hence reducing the need to rationalize the choices.

After-school activities are a great example of this. You may have a great meal planned for the evening after soccer or dance and then the traffic is worse than usual, or practice ran 20 minutes over (Excuses!), and now you are scrambling to get homework and dinner done before bath and bedtime. Pack healthy, small finger food meals at the beginning of the week and bring them with you in the morning (works well if you have a fridge at the office). Now, both you and the kids have an opportunity to eat healthy before practice even begins, or although not ideal, it is a portable healthy option on the road. This will reduce the possible stressors after practice that are only remedied by a drive through the fast food parking lot.

Journaling is another way to find those emotional triggers that have the potential to create the biggest road blocks to your overall health and wellness, and map out remedies to address the issues before they occur. Failing to plan can certainly lead to an inevitable plan to fail. One way that I do this (when I know that I am having emotional triggers and may be tempted to find the nearest cookie cake and just dig in) is changing the activity to something that will positively motivate me. I have always loved window shopping. Now that we have so many shops online, you can do this anywhere, anytime! What I do is look at an item that I would love to add to my wardrobe and take a snapshot of the item. It can motivate me to stay on course with the anticipation of wearing the outfit in the future, and this small insignificant strategy does wonders to encourage me. Instead of buying this pint of ice cream, I could put the money toward this incredible new blazer for the upcoming "Sweata Weatha"!

Depression and Trauma

Sometimes things occur in our lives such as anxiety, depression or other mental disorders that create more opportunity to stress or emotionally eat. Again, find the triggers and work on solutions that will reduce the occurrences. If your depression or anxiety is presently being managed with medications, it is possible that they can slow down the progress with your weight loss plan. Talk with your provider about what your plan for weight loss management entails, and seek advice on some alternative medications. I know it sounds redundant, but in reality, this method can be used in so many ways. It is essentially the preparation that allows for the greatest success, which we will get to momentarily! There are times where some roadblocks are associated with past childhood traumas such as emotional, physical or even sexual abuse. There are some individuals that will hide or protect themselves with food and weight gain. This can be a major roadblock or rationalization to long term weight loss and wellness. If this is the case, it may require more aggressive strategies such as counseling to address the underlying issues. If not addressed, they will certainly lead to major setbacks on your road to health and recovery. You want to be a healthy you, through and through. There are issues that create road-blocks so working on strategies now can reduce the reactive choices when the stressor occurs.

Everyone rationalizes, but what you say to yourself and what you ultimately choose to do will create the environment for success or failure. The choice? Well, that is yours, of course! Remember, excuses are the easiest solution to the problem, because they take very little effort. What you want most will take effort and will-power to achieve. Reaching your long-term goals successfully is not for the faint at heart, but it can be achieved by anyone who will put his/her mind to it!

CHAPTER 6

Expectation: The Ultimate Shell Game

Online dating. It is probably one of the best examples that I can use to describe how different our expectations are to the reality that we face. Most individuals who have attempted to use this platform to find the "love of their life" will tell you it is not as easy as the advertisements lead you to believe. Kissing a few frogs before finding your prince? Well, welcome to the swamp my friends! Just as social media prompts you to portray the absolute best of yourself and anything less will simply not do, the online dating scene is where the professionals go to play. Don't get me wrong, I think that this platform has its advantages to finding someone that is like-minded and may even enjoy similar hobbies, but many are so critical of their true selves that they will simply succumb to the peer pressure to dress up their profile with a bit of exaggerated details. It doesn't help that as a society we have fallen victim to the expectation that what we experience and view on television should obviously happen in real life. Not sure what I am referring to? Two lonely individuals in the heart of New York, longing to meet their soul mate, happen upon each other with a little rendition of "You've Got Mail." For our younger readers, what about the reality TV series that portrays the lives of bounty hunters, alligator wranglers, and even 5 sisters and a mother's every-day life, as fast-paced, incredibly rich, even glamourous, making the viewer long for a life just remotely similar. Are the lives of Dog, Shelby, and even the Kardashian's really anymore incredible than, let's say, the lives of teachers, bankers, and yes, even nurse practitioners? Yet, we have set DVRs, moved schedules around to see the newest episodes, and even deferred opportunities to hang out with family and friends just to get a glimpse of our favorite reality series.

In our day-to-day lives, there seems to be an incredible discrepancy between our expectations and the reality that we experience, a shell game of sorts. A great example of the difference between expectations and reality is when I have a chance to visit with one of our Obstetrical patients in the latter part of their pregnancy. I will often ask them if they have everything ready for the baby. What is so fascinating to me is that my first-time Mothers have everything painted, put together, packed up for the hospital and freshly washed, while my seasoned mothers roll in with one in tow and hair in a messy bun telling me they haven't started shopping for the new bundle of joy yet. I instruct them about the symptoms of postpartum depression and the potential triggers that may be involved when experiencing this condition. There are a few that will give me this condescending look like, "Really?!? I don't think you need to worry yourself about that!" Their expectation is that their transition into parenthood will be like an opening number of a musical on Broadway. I believe they envision the welcome home scene for the newborn to look something like this: the sound of music plays softly in the background as the baby wakes in the morning for their diaper change and first meal of the day. Maybe even a few bluebirds chirp away as the baby sits quietly swaddled in the crib. During the night, around 3 am, after sleeping for 5 hours, the baby is heard cooing from the crib, indicating the need for a quick diaper change and feeding before settling down again for 4 to 5 hours of sound sleep! WAKE UP! Fast forward to the delivery, recovery, and discharge to their homes, where they realize that the only music to their ears is the sound of the microwave in motion sterilizing the bottles. The melody of a newborn's screeching cry that could be heard as far as the next neighborhood, that cannot be quieted by anything but possibly a blow-dryer or a vacuum cleaner, becomes an all-familiar tune. These same parents show up for the post-partum visit resembling someone that may have gone 3 rounds in a closed ring with Mike Tyson just looking for an ear to bite!

They realize that the expectations they had going into parenthood are quite different from the reality of dealing with a newborn's demands day in and day out.

Expectations for those attempting weight loss and wellness are quite similar to our reality TV viewers, online daters and even our new parents. Often, those that desire weight loss may proceed into a weight loss plan with the expectation that they will go from a tight size 16 to looking like a Runway Model in less than 6 weeks! You may even have fallen prey to the many fad eating plans out there that give the dieter the expectation that they will lose 10 inches in the first 7 days of the eating plan-all the while eating cheesecake every night for dessert! There are false expectations related to getting into physical shape with a plethora of options out there selling quick results with minimal effort.

In all seriousness, we (and I mean me) have all fallen prey to the tantalizing infomercials that draw us in under the premise of immediate results within the first 3 days. I have bought an abdominal roller, HIIT fitness videos, dance videos, and a special 90-day program, the list is truly endless! It sounds so incredible and who wouldn't believe that you can really lose 30 pounds in 6 weeks simply by doing a particular exercise regimen for 15 minutes every day? I have mentioned this before. When I am counseling a patient on weight loss (whether it is metabolic in nature or just situation/emotional stressors) I ask them a rhetorical question. "If I were to drive from Louisiana to California and in Texas decide to turn around, where exactly am I?" I'm still in Texas! When you make the decision to achieve your weight loss goals and a lifestyle of improved wellness, you are not already at the finish line. In fact, the gun hasn't even gone off yet beginning the race! You have, at that point, just decided to RUN the race, but there are several additional things to consider before jumping in and setting yourself at the line.

A dear friend of mine, in fact she is like family, has recently gone through a very difficult surgery and recovery period, and she handled the recovery like a champ! One of the side effects of the medications she was taking at the time is an increased risk of kidney stones. Unfortunately, she developed several stones that required a stent to be inserted in the ureters to help pass the remaining particles. It was a very difficult time. She had a significant amount of pain, and she was very sick from the side effects of the stent and medications. Acknowledging the condition was very frustrating and even a bit discouraging for her. I texted her one morning and sent her a short message about my very brief stent on the high school track team. I really joined the track team because I was dating someone on the boy's track team, which should have been a red flag, as this sport was not my cup of tea, but such is life! So, the coach signed me up for the distance running. I was assigned the 1600 meter which is essentially a mile. You need to know something here. I hate to run. In fact, the only time you will find me running, is if someone is chasing me with either a sharp tool or knife and unless it is significant, I probably wouldn't run from that either! Anyway, what I found through this experience is that it was really easy to go up to the line and get set. In fact, the first lap that I ran was not very difficult. On the second lap, I started to get a little winded, but I was still holding my own. Now on the 3rd lap, typically on the back half of the track there is a phenomenon known as the bear hug. You have this sensation that this "bear" jumps on your back, wraps his big arms around you, and you are left with no other option but to carry him the rest of the way. It becomes extremely more taxing just to get around the curve, and you feel as if finishing this race is just not in the cards for you.

After getting through the 3rd lap and beginning the last lap of the race, you meet up with something called, "your second wind." It helps you to finish the race. As a side note, unfortunately I am not able to speak to this from direct experience. I have no idea what the second wind feels like, as the only thing I gleaned from distance running was severe muscle cramps to my sides! She appreciated the example, but when you are in the fight, dueling it out, YOU feel each and every blow that is being thrown, and it makes staying in the fight very difficult.

You see, the only way to complete the race is to train, practice, and RUN the race. The expectation that weight loss will come easy and without any obstacles is simply a false expectation. Ultimately this will lead to a failure in accomplishing the task that you set before yourself. It all comes down to hard work, plain and simple. I have a saying I use often with my patients; if it flops like a fish, smells like a fish, and jumps like a fish......well, it's a fish! If the program that you are contemplating sounds too easy to do, there is no hard work involved to obtain significant results, and it won't require any sacrifice, now you can consider running in the opposite direction!

There are a few old adages out there about hard work. Calvin Coolidge once said, "All growth depends upon activity. There is no development physically or intellectually without effort, and effort means work." We live in a world where we are expecting microwave results when the only way to achieve these results is through a slow-cooker process. Simply put, without realistic goals that you actively work toward achieving, the cute outfits you are picking out online are just that, cute outfits. Developing realistic goals is essential, but you have to have an Aha! Moment; an epiphany that what you do each day and every day to reach your goals is more important than the goals themselves. I am not minimizing the need for goals, absolutely not! However, you can spend hours drawing up an exercise routine, reading books on weight loss, and even binge on Pinterest for awesome low carb recipes (been there, done ALL of this), but without the motion, activity, and forward movement to implement these goals, it, my friend, was a waste of precious time.

Thomas Edison, who may have failed more than he succeeded, had the mentality to never give up and always worked hard, said this, "The three great essentials to achieve anything worthwhile are, first, hard work: second, stick-to-itiveness; third, common sense." I love this adage because frankly, we could all use more stick-to-itiveness. Hard work is what sets the goal in motion, but without a resolve to maintain the motion, the goal is just a quick flash in the pan. You have seen this happen to people around you. In fact, you could have been the one they were making bets on! They come in after a month-long holiday celebration, or, in Louisiana, they have hit the king cakes hard, I mean really hard, and they roll in on Ash Wednesday stating to all that will lend an ear, they are giving up sweets, all sugars and they are going full blown 1000 calorie a day keto! That's when all bets are on and fellow employees are secretly taking odds on how long she will make it until she hits the robin eggs in the Easter Candy aisle. (Ok, this may have happened to me once, ok maybe twice, whatever let's move on!) Having Stick-to-itiveness means that even when someone brings those amazing donuts for Friday breakfast at work, or your husband's birthday comes up and you go out to have a celebratory meal, you, my friend, have to reach back into the dark corners of your mind where those goals are sitting and not budge. Remain steadfast in what you ultimately want to accomplish. Remember, making our expectations something we can stick to contributes to our long-term success. Is it easy? (Insert a Disney villain laugh here) No! It's not easy to avoid the candy, donuts, or the second helping when it is a mac-daddy meal, but if you can train the brain to realize it is a short window of satisfaction but a long road to recovery, then you will be able to start achieving those amazing goals. Remember, we are always trying to keep that emotional monster in check, and if we can implement proactive strategies, it provides less opportunity to reactively choose.

Common sense should be plain and simple, but unfortunately this is not the case. Make sure that you actively evoke your common sense or set the expectations wisely when trying to develop goals and implement them. If you decide that you are only going to eat lean meats and greens for 1 month and you aren't fond of greens, then this may be a goal that does not bode well in your favor. When you go out with friends, use some common sense when looking for a place to meet, greet, and eat. Don't pick a fried food establishment where the only thing remotely healthy on the menu is a pack of mustard. When is the best time to go grocery shopping? When you have just eaten a healthy but fulfilling meal. Why? If you are famished, your stomach will hijack your brain and tell you that you need all of those things on the shelves or in the frozen food section (not the healthiest options) simply because you are riding the *hangry* train to *regretville*. Many times, when I need things in the grocery, I walk in and forego the buggy or basket. Why? Again, use common sense. When you are walking up and down aisles looking for a particular item like your Korean paste but you pass the potato chip aisle on your way, you may be inclined to throw a few bags into the buggy. Yeah, you could still grab a bag of chips and manage to carry your paste too, but there isn't much more that you will be able to juggle without the potential of having the store manager call overhead for a clean-up on aisle 4! We talked earlier about proactively planning. This is a must for stick-to-itiveness and common sense. When you pack a bag of good snack options and a healthy lunch, you are less inclined to succumb to the reactive opportunities that will arise during the day. Our office is the worst when it comes to temptations in the breakroom (sounds like a blues song!). King cake season! It's nothing to have a king cake delivered to the office 2 to 3 times in a week, or 2 to 3 times a day for that matter. Drug reps are notorious for bringing an awesome dessert to go with the meal, so we can sit a little bit longer in the break room to hear their spiel. Domestic executives (a.k.a. Stay at home mothers), need to ensure that the snacks you have in the pantry or fridge for the little ones aren't creating temptations that are too much to bear. They need healthy choices too, and when you only have those options available, making the right choice is so much easier. To think that you can buy sweet treats for the family and you will be able to withstand the temptation is not using the common sense you need to make this work. No, you shouldn't have the ding dongs parked in your pantry as a sweet treat for the little ones on a Friday! If your emotional monster happens to be on a tangent, then you have stacked the deck in his favor! Preparation and proactive planning will always provide a mechanism to avoid the pitfalls and assist you in creating an environment to reach your goals.

One of my favorite adages by Vince Lombardi simply says this, "Those at the top of the mountain didn't fall there." (It took everything inside of me not to put an exclamation at the end of that statement because I could see someone screaming this at the top of the mountain!) When you see a friend on social media posting before and after shots of where they were and what they look like now, do you really think that happened in 30 days? Please! Social media is the epitome of showing only the best of you, not the rest of you. We see a few gym monkeys on snap-chat or maybe pumping the iron in the gym and think well, it really can't be that hard to look like that? What these guys have achieved was nothing short of hard work, dedication, and yes, they may have used a specific eating plan or program to obtain the goals, but there were goals established and achieved, none the less.

My son lives in Colorado. He has been there for several years now, and for a few years he lived in Breckenridge. The altitude is well over 9,000 feet above sea level. We visited during the summer one year. It was amazing, and he brought us on some hikes to see lakes at the top of the mountains. Just to get to the part where the trail actually began was a hike. With minimum training and little exercise at the time, we (meaning me) expected to walk up this mountain without any resistance, obstacles, or discomfort. Without adequate preparation, we expected to reach the top of the mountain. Climbing physical mountains is certainly not easy without adequate preparation, and when you are trying to tame the emotional monster and climb the mountain in front of you to reach your goal, it, my friend, will not be easy either. You WILL have to prepare. You WILL confront frequent obstacles along the way, and it WON'T always "feel" great. When we fail to prepare, we will be prepared to fail!

Again, this is not rocket science, this is common sense. One of the easiest ways to implement successful strategies is to ensure that, with your overall end goal, you have several short-term goals that will create positive pushing-points toward ultimately achieving the goal. As we alluded to in the last chapter, several short wins can create an unstoppable momentum for you to reach the goal you set. Maybe your initial goals are to stop drinking soda and change to water or healthier options. You may decide a great short win is to ensure that you prep your snacks for the day before you start doing full meal prepping. The point is, forward motion is still forward. It is still getting you closer to the end result. When I counsel my patients who have a significant amount of weight to lose, I ask them what short term weight loss expectation they want to establish first. A pound a week? 20 pounds in the next 2 months? Set a realistic expectation to create a platform for the greatest success.

Sometimes looking at the big picture can be overwhelming but when you hone in on a fragment of it and focus your efforts on those short wins, when you step back, you have made progress. Another thing I will share with my patients is simply this, if you lose a pound a week, which is very feasible, when you see me in the office one year later, you will have lost 52 pounds. Their eyes light up because they realize that the short-term goal is very possible, but creates amazing long-term results. It's a must to set realistic expectations. Everyone, and I mean everyone, has an expectation for themselves. Often, we make assumptions that the expectations set are realistic and reasonable, and when they are not achieved, this can be very devastating to some. When trying to achieve weight loss and become healthier, without good realistic expectations, if not careful, we can create an environment for failure.

Here is the deal. You cannot expect to NEVER have a slip-up or cravings for your favorite foods; this is going to happen. It is what you do to prepare for those times that will truly create the foundation for your success. If you slipped and had a donut during the morning staff meeting, that doesn't justify an all-out binge on French fries and triple decker burgers for lunch! What intervention did you implement to ensure that you immediately got back on your plan? One thing I know with certainty is this, you will have emotional highs and lows. This is not going away. What you are trying to implement are strategies to avoid the pitfalls that come with the highs and the lows. You are trying to redevelop your conditional response to the emotions you have. Say what, Kelly?!

Essentially, you want to retrain the brain to think differently when you experience that emotional high or low and change your expectations. When you adequately prepare, you are establishing new rules and guidelines that you want your brain to follow, and over time, you can create positive responses to the inevitable emotional rollercoaster of life. It is impossible to have big wins 100% of the time, and society has created the expectation that anything short of this is not considered success. When you set unrealistic expectations, you are actually creating an opportunity for the emotional monster to have a dance party on your goals and overall success. This can actually create more highs and lows than typically experienced by making it hard to achieve some form of everyday success.

First, we must become clear on what our long and short-term goals are so our expectations are realistic.

- How much overall weight do I want to lose?
- What period of time will I allow myself to reach my weight loss goal?
- What strategies do I need to implement to meet my short and overall goals?

Obviously, the specifics to the goals will be different for everyone, but the goal-setting is always the same. Make healthy, realistic goals and create achievable strategies and choices to obtain your overall weight loss and improved health. You need to take some time, sit down uninterrupted, and ask yourself:

- What are my overall goals?
- What do I want to ultimately achieve?
- What does the ideal picture of my health and weight loss wellness look like?
- Have I developed any unrealistic expectations to reach the goals I have set?

These are questions that only you can answer. Again, you must have that epiphany moment like I did on that scale in my friend's condo.

Other things to consider when setting expectations: Take a historical journey back in time to your successes and failures with weight loss and wellness. Really evaluate what worked well for you and what needs to be thrown into the scrap pile. There is a saying that goes something like this, "When you don't aim for the bull's eye, you will hit that spot every time." Keep what has worked for you in the past, even if it may need a little tweaking, but trash the methods that opened the door for obstacles or even failure. Fad diets are the worst because they create the mindset that you will be able to quickly achieve your goal and maintain the loss long-term. Often, they create a yo-yo like effect for individuals, and ultimately, you not only gain the weight previously lost, but you also manage to find additional weight along the way. You know, I see many patients who suffer with obesity and decide to have permanent weight loss surgery, losing an incredible amount of weight during the process. These same individuals show up a few years later having gained most of the weight back. Why? No matter what you use to achieve the goal, if your mind-set and emotional reactions to food are not addressed, your long-term goals for wellness and weight loss will be but a brief flash in the pan.

Create an atmosphere for constant evaluation.

- What worked?
- What didn't work?
- What can be revised and changed a little and still be utilized with success?
- Were there unrealistic expectations that I had. If so, what changes can I make to prevent this in the future?

If you are an avid sports fan, you know when you watch a team, especially a great team, being coached, they are always being evaluated.

- What worked?
- Has man on man worked better than zone?
- Will they blitz this time?
- Are they covering my wide-outs?

Yes, I do like football! The coaches are looking at defense and offense. What do I need to do to shore up my defense, (combat reactive choices) and what are some offensive moves that will help us to obtain the win? (Increase water intake or start exercising at least 2-3 times a week).

In addition, make sure to incorporate an accountability measure or an accountability partner who will actively and positively provide feedback to help you obtain your overall goal. Someone who will give you realistic feedback, providing an environment for constructive feedback and opportunities for improvement. Great players, inevitably have an amazing coach pushing them to excel, driving their strengths, and giving them support to work on their opportunities. Carefully choose the voice of reason in your life. You need a realistic voice giving you necessary, timely feedback. Avoid the pie-in-the-sky friends, or even worse, avoid those individuals that may have the Chicken Little mentality that the sky is falling!

One of the most effective tools for goal-setting is the SMART goals. This is an acronym that simply stands for Specific, Measurable, Attainable, Relevant, and Time Bound goals. What would this look like for weight loss and overall health and wellness? Specific goals (I want to lose 25 pounds), Measurable (I will do a weekly weigh-in), Attainable (losing 1 pound a week with a specific eating plan I can reach this goal in this amount of time), Relevant (am I achieving a goal that will benefit me, and is it realistic?), and Time bound (I will lose the 25 pounds in a period of 4-5 months). Make sure the expectations you have set are motivational to you, are attainable, and put in writing. It's one thing to say you want to lose 25 pounds. It's a whole other thing to put that goal down on a piece of paper with additional strategies notated. Your action plan will ultimately determine your greatest success. Without vision, the people will perish, but without a map, you will just stay lost! Map out your plan. Take time to look ahead for potential pit-falls (birthdays, special events, etc.), and pencil in work-arounds for the obstacles before you even begin.

We have covered a lot relative to Expectations. Make sure when you are working on this portion of your PREP FOR IT program that you ensure these are YOUR Expectations, not your husband's, mother's, or friend's expectations for you in this weight loss and wellness process. Make sure that you don't have a false expectation or self-image. We ALWAYS see ourselves worse than others see us. Be kind to yourself. Be positive to becoming the new you, and of course, embrace the process. There is always a process if you want the prize.

CHAPTER 7

Preparation: Living in Hurricane Alley

If you are someone who can't wait to get to the end of the movie to find out "who dunit?" then we are getting a little closer to Inspector Clouseau's big reveal. In order to provide an environment that will allow you to finally curtail that emotional monster that has made 104 YOU Boulevard his home address, we need to ensure that your preparation for weight loss and overall wellness is packed full of useful tools, timely resources, and a thought-out process that will lead to your success.

I live in south Louisiana the land of alligators, crawfish, and hurricanes, and that isn't just the alcoholic beverage either. Hurricane season, believe it or not, runs from July through November, literally half of our calendar year. Generally, these months are non-eventful, and life strums along as usual. However, when the water temperature warms up just right in the Gulf of Mexico, hurricane season is not for the faint at heart. We experienced a devastating season in 2005, when Hurricane Katrina made landfall on the shores of Mississippi and Louisiana, affecting millions of families through the loss of loved ones, homes, as well as affecting our laid-back culture that we are so accustomed to living. We didn't evacuate for the storm. A lot of people didn't. We were fortunate, but there were many who were significantly affected. What is so ironic, is that when July rolls around there is a plethora of information to help those in Hurricane Alley implement preparation strategies. Seriously, tons of information is broadcasted through mail-outs, emergency preparedness notifications on the radio and television, flyers sent out by the utility company, and even drills that are done by medical facilities and emergency services. Many painstaking measures take place to ensure that those living in this area are well informed and prepared. However, the onus still falls on the individual, and that's where trouble finds a great place to have a party. Inevitably, when there is mass notification of an impending storm in the Gulf, there will always be those who find themselves ill-prepared, scouring the home for flashlights, candles, and playing cards, emptying out the nearest Grocery or Hardware store of bottled water, batteries, and bread. They may even wind-up parking in line, for hours on end, at the gas station only to get to the pump and find out that the well has run dry. All because they waited to prepare. They are typically left with limited resources, very little choices for supplies, or even left without having some vital tools for the stirring storm in the gulf. Others opt to stay despite the governmental recommendations to evacuate and weather the storm and all that it may entail. What you do ahead of time to prepare for the impending storm will ultimately determine what affect the storm has in your life.

Consider your weight loss and wellness goals like a great storm brewing in the gulf. You know it's time to batten down the hatches and start making better choices and putting some serious plans in place, but you inevitably find yourself scurrying through the fast food drive thru, attempting to get some form of a healthy option (news flash!! Fast Food restaurants are not an option when you are really trying to achieve a healthier you). Don't get me wrong, there is nothing wrong with a chicken sandwich, (on occasion!) but let's face it, if you want to achieve significant weight loss and overall health, you will need to put some serious action plans and preparation in place.

It is crucial to provide ample time to identify the need, make appropriate preparations, and execute the plan efficiently. We have gone through the PREP FOR IT process thus far, alluding to the Perception, Rationalization, and Expectation as very important components to the process, but Preparation is the glue that holds this system in place. What you do to sit down and formulate the plan to gain control of the emotional monster in your life, how you decide to take him down and keep him in check, really boils down to planning, planning, and oh, did I mention planning?

Kelly, I get it, I need to plan!

Well, duh! Planning is not just about the process that we are going to use to execute the goals that we have decided to set in place; it is about anticipating the ups and downs on a day-to-day basis, what will be the counter measure to ensure we do not derail out of the terminal, and how we will execute the preparation weekly to ensure that those goals are in fact, achieved. Preparation in respect to our program, is designed to help establish a weekly routine that will allow us to plan our weekly meals and snacks, set aside time to actually prepare them in order to establish food as a function in our lives and consider any possible pitfalls that we could encounter within the next week.

Food prep is not a novel or new concept. There are many videos, books, and media resources that will give you information on food prepping. So, what makes our food prep system any different? We wanted to make food prep easy to accomplish, not over-bearing and mundane, and we wanted to equip our readers with recipes that would knock their socks off! It's one thing to be on an eating plan to help reach our weight loss and wellness goals, but it's a whole other level to have foods that make your co-workers slip on their saliva in the breakroom. Food prepping shouldn't be boring, it shouldn't be bland, and it shouldn't be bothersome. It should be the plan that gets you to your end goal, while allowing you to enjoy the process, smell the roses, and eat great food along the way! Going all the way back to the chapter on my testimony, I needed to go back to a system that had worked well for me, one that I was most successful using. What was easy to follow, but flavorful to stick with? What made food a function and not an occasion? What made me feel satiated and not deprived in the process? What exercise programs did I thoroughly enjoy, and what activities did I loathe participating in? (That will always be running for me, FYI!)

Some individuals have negative feelings about prepping. I don't have time. I work too much. It's hard to have the time when the kids are in the kitchen with me. I don't like leftovers (News flash, they are not leftovers; you haven't eaten it yet!) I don't like microwaving my food. Really the list can go on, but ultimately, we need to look at these comments for what they are.... Rationalization (excuses!) as to why yet another program will not work for them. Until you can man or woman up and say, "You know what? I NEED to make the time to prepare for the week ahead, so I can have the best outcome possible," then there will always be an activity, family members, or financial issues that will stand in your way.

When you start planning your food prep, you need to evaluate a few key points to ensure your greatest success. Let us start with the most obvious. Can I cook?? If you have a difficult time boiling an egg, this will be a factor (not an obstacle) in preparing to food prep. We tried to offer recipes that were not overly difficult to replicate in addition to having amazing flavor. Of course, you will need to know a few essentials (how to chop an onion, how to take down a cauliflower head, and what par-boiling means) to facilitate a smooth prep process. Our PREP FOR IT Essentials 101 video provided with the book, allows the novice prepper to learn basic kitchen functions, with easy step-by-step instructions. It's one thing to tell someone what to do, (Go fish for food) but it's a whole other level to actually teach the basics to become a successful angler! So, knowledge is power my friend, and when you know the process, kicking the emotional monster to the curb will be far easier to do. The essentials video is meant to provide an avenue for those who may not feel incredibly comfortable in the kitchen or around utensils and would like step-by-step guidance to successfully meal-prep and plan for the week. For those "seasoned" in the kitchen, the book will provide all of the necessary resources to get the job done quite effectively.

Do I have the financial capability to food prep?

Historically, organic food options were always more expensive, making healthy eating and living harder to obtain. However, since more individuals are looking for healthier options, it has forced some of the larger supermarkets to buck up and provide healthier food options at an affordable cost to the consumer. The best way to figure out if you have enough money to food prep, is to go back in your banking account for the last 3 months and add up all of the expenditures on coffee, fast food lunches, and dinners out. Once when I was doing an evaluation of our finances, I realized I had spent over $500 a month on specialty coffee! Don't get me wrong, I love a great cappuccino, but do you realize that what was spent on coffee would easily cover the cost of food prepping plus some of the supplies, and I would be healthy in the process? Quite simply, you cannot afford to avoid food prep based on financial restrictions alone. You are doing yourself a disservice if you do not invest in your overall health and weight loss and see it as a true investment into your future. Much like you view your 401K or IRA. We tried to set up the weekly recipes to be able to use foods in more than one way, to avoid overspending and wasting the resources you have available to you. Another thing to consider is doubling the recipes and freezing your food prep when applicable since many large grocery stores will offer bulk meats and veggies for a discounted price. Take advantage of the sales at your local grocery and what will work in your recipe artillery for that week. The great thing about the recipes and resources is it does most of the planning for you, so really, it's about time management, both from the perspective of shopping and the actual prepping itself.

Do I have the resources at home to food prep for the week?

When you evaluate what tools of the trade are already available in your kitchen to make this work, there are a few essentials that make this job much easier to accomplish but certainly not impossible. Many of the tools that we use to make prep much easier are things like mechanical peelers, parchment paper, aluminum pans, vegetable scooper, a great chopping/paring knife, and really great storage containers. Most of the other supplies are awesome to have but are not necessary to reach your end goal. Make sure and do an inventory of your kitchen supplies and equipment, then make a list of the must-haves to get the job done.

- Do I have a great stew pot?
- How many cookie sheets do I have?
- Do I have a great knife for cutting veggies and meat?
- Do I have a slow cooker or food processor?

We have provided a list of equipment essentials in the supplemental workbook to make this process easier to complete. Please don't use the lack of resources as a limitation for you to obtain a healthier version of yourself. This is an investment that will start to pay immediate dividends and will continue to pay out in your future.

I just don't have the time over the weekend to spend 2-3 hours in the kitchen. I work all week and have activities I bring the children to during the weekend. I know this sounds like a valid reason for avoiding meal preparation in your life, but unfortunately again, this is just Rationalization (cough, excuses, cough, cough). When I work with patients in the office to help them establish a good weight-loss plan in their life, the most common reason for their lack of planning and success is, "You just don't know how busy my life is, Kelly. I work 12-hour days, 5 days a week, and I am just exhausted when I get home."

Let's put a different spin on this. If you work 12-hour days, 5 days a week, then having a meal already prepared in the fridge for you to simply take out, warm up and enjoy will actually offer you more time at home to recuperate before you need to get up and do it all again! Additionally, you would avoid feeling overwhelmed, which could lead to making poor food choices and allowing the emotional monster to do the happy dance all over you as you cruise through the drive thru for some fried chicken! Please! This particular factor is what causes most individuals to rationalize their way out of a healthier life style. I travel too much, the kids are in too many activities, the dog ate my food prep containers! Rationalizing why you are not able to take the time to meal prep hurts only one individual along the way…you. Again, you have to have the aha moment when you say, enough is enough to the emotional monster and take your life back to finally obtain a healthier version of you.

Getting back to hurricane preparedness. I did some research on an organization that is in the business of preparing, the Red Cross. Most people think the Red Cross is about providing for the tragedy after it occurs, not helping individuals to prevent it, but that is actually not the case. The Red Cross has a video on its website titled, "Steps to Prep." It focuses on 3 main points to help individuals prepare for impending disasters. The first step is, Get a Kit. I love this! They recommend putting a kit together before any impending disasters like flashlights, water, non-perishable food items, etc. In PREP FOR IT terms, getting a kit would be the equivalent of making sure you have the tools, recipes, seasonings, and ingredients to do the job before you get into the kitchen and start making the mess.

We wanted to make the prep process super easy. Our goal was to put together a short 6-week meal prep that would provide our readers, a turn-key option that minimized the need to do plenty of research and planning and to focus more on the PREP acronyms for a greater opportunity of long-term success. If you are stressing about preparing, then you will be prepared to stress eat, and nobody has got time for all of that! So, we have compiled several of our favorite recipes that are great right out of the oven, or even when reheated (this is important in relation to food as a function and having easy and quick accessibility). We have also put together the grocery lists and options to consider for snacking when you "feel the need" hitting you! Other than going shopping for the food and actually making it, we have tried to do most of the planning for you.

The second step in their process is, Make a Plan. Well, hellloooo!?! I think we have beat this point into the ground, but for sake of the Red Cross steps, having a plan allows you to avoid the pitfalls, the knee-jerk responses and keeps the emotional monster in check. This isn't just for food preparation, it's for snack and event planning, exercise routines and how to get back on track when you derail the train. Although we have put together a

6-week starter course to assist you in getting this train out of the station, it is imperative that you make plans for the "what ifs," "so then what's," and worst of all, "now what's??" moments in your life. Your plan has to be more than just getting the grocery list, snack list, and your kitchen prepared. It needs to be a plan of attack, day in and day out, when the emotional highs and lows occur, and we all know this part of the equation is a given.

The final step in the Red Cross, Steps to Prep, is Be Informed. Yes, be informed! Do the research, read the book, look at the resources you have available, keep up with things that will inevitably make you more prepared for the storm. Again, I cannot stress this enough, this is NOT rocket science. It is good old-fashioned stick-to-itiveness that we discussed previously, and that is the difference maker to be prepared. To stay, in the know, we created Prep4it.com to provide numerous additional resources that go beyond your 6 week PREP for it plan.

The American Psychological Association has an article posted on their website on "How to emotionally prepare for a hurricane" that was written by Raymond F. Hanbury PhD. and Eva D. Sivan PhD. Out of all of the things we have discussed thus far, I feel this is the most important component of this puzzle. Remember what got you here. The emotional monster wreaking havoc in your life. Taking every extreme emotion and issue you have in your day-to-day life and create an environment of emotional and comfort eating that caused you to spiral out of control. Don't feed the beast!

Do you know why this is so important? Because feeding the beast makes it stronger, gives it more control in your life, and causes you to feel helpless. There is a reason why there are signs in National parks telling you not to feed the wildlife. First, it makes them rely on you for their food. When you feed into what the emotional monster is doing in your life, you are creating an environment of neediness and a conditional response that only hurts you in the long run. Secondly, it makes the animal more aggressive. It's not enough that you throw a few nuts or a banana out the window when you see an animal while driving through the park; enough is never enough! First, they make their way to the side of the road, then your car, and before you know it, they are trying to open the door to get a little too close for your comfort! When my brother was a tween, my mother and father took him on a vacation to New Brunswick, Texas and they drove through a wildlife park, where it was encouraged to feed the animals. The absolute best part of this trip for my dad was when the ostrich came up to the window and not only ate food out of my brother's hand, but proceeded to stick his long neck into the car to get up close and personal. Well needless to say, Ronnie quickly made his way onto my mother's lap (who was driving the car) leaving Dad in stitches in the back seat! Your emotional monster is not any different; enough will never be enough! He will start with a few small episodes and then eventually, throw the routine temper tantrums in your life, making you succumb to the king cakes, donuts, and cookies of the world; don't do it!

As I have digressed, back to our article. The article offered readers tips on strengthening themselves emotionally before having to go through a hurricane. It addresses the uncertainty the massive influx of information about the storm, and what affects the storm can have in your life. A few ways they suggested to emotionally prepare include, have a plan and implement it.

What in the world? Kelly, they want you to have a plan too?

Yep, pretty much. Your plan is the biggest weapon against the emotional monster and the rollercoaster he is attempting to strap you to. What is so ironic is, take a guess who they referenced for making a plan? You got it! The Red Cross! Preparing with a plan in advance, reduces your anxiety and creates the proactive planning concept that ultimately reduces reactive choices.

Another step they alluded to is getting the facts. This is just funny now. Do your research, know what works and doesn't work for you. Making sure that you understand what you will be doing so that the actual implementation is not your obstacle. The basic 6-week prep course and Essential 101 video are a few specific resources to help you put this plan in place and provide the means and facts to make the process a little easier. The Essentials 101 video is probably my favorite. The video not only teaches you about the different utensils, but also how to put them into practice. How many times have you pushed your buggy through the kitchen tool section of the store and wondered, what is this gadget even used for? Many of the things that we recommend are basic tools of the trade that will definitely provide some shortcuts to the prepping process (go to prep4it.com to check out the video).

The next step, Make Connections. This is an incredible point. You need to have some accountability. Your proactive planning should help you day to day, but having a trusted individual in your life who can tell you the great things you need to hear to fuel the fire, and then address the more concerning issues is crucial for your success. Is it an absolute? Not necessarily, but having that person to create the glass-check moments, can ease some burdens and avoid potential pitfalls along the way.

Another step in the process, is to stay healthy and to quote, "A healthy lifestyle including proper diet, exercise and rest-is your best defense again any threat. A healthy body can have a positive impact on your thoughts and emotions, enabling you to make better decisions and better deal with the hurricane's uncertainties." Seriously, I can't make this up! Your best weapon against the emotional monster may be preparation, but your best defense to ensure your uncertainties are minimized, is a healthy self. By implementing the strategies we have talked about, you literally are creating mechanisms that will reverse the vicious cycle that was discussed earlier in the book.

The last point discussed, in the American Psychological Association article, is to maintain a hopeful outlook. They recommend drawing on past experiences that have successfully managed past challenges to help through the current storm. Wow! Enough said. Find what works, and stick with it, paint the barn door until the paint sticks, and don't reinvent the wheel you may have done a successful wheelie on in the past. However, the opposite side of the coin that ensures you will have a hopeful outlook, is to make sure to not overdramatize the pitfalls and the bumps YOU WILL experience along the way. Eating something you are not supposed to is going to happen. Making reactive choices during the course of a day is going to happen. What you do after these events occur is a game changer. Seriously, do not sweat the small stuff. So, are you saying it's ok to eat the donuts in the break room?

NOPE! NADA! WHAT YOU TALKIN' ABOUT, WILLIS?! But if you made a reactive decision at breakfast, don't let it sabotage the rest of the day for you. Pull your bootstraps up and get back on the band wagon for the rest of the day.

As always, we want to make sure you take time to ask yourself some questions that will help to formulate the most successful plan for you. This is not a cookie cutter program. It's a process to find what works best for you and a method that will help you to achieve the end-goal. In the next chapter, we are going to get into the nuts and bolts of the program and teach what food prepping can look like for you. We will go through the main meals of the day, snacks, pitfalls, and week in review. But before we get there, take a few minutes to really go through these questions, do the homework and research, maybe even write your answers down and review them so you have a better understanding of what your plan will look like. We referenced this earlier in the book; by failing to plan, you are essentially planning to fail. Give yourself everything you need to be successful and with the stick-to-itiveness, you will accomplish weight loss and overall wellness in your life.

CHAPTER 8

What's The Plan, Stan? The PREP FOR IT Program

Vacations are meant to be relaxing, a time of unwinding and rebooting your mental computer so that you have the potential to function as a better version of yourself. For some, it is simply as easy as stuffing a few things in a bag, packing the toothbrush, filling up the car, and figuring everything else out on the way to your destination. Reservations? Nah! We will figure it out when we get there! While for others, (enter Kelly, stage left!) we will go through months of planning, researching, surfing the web to find the coolest, neatest things to do and making sure that…. every…. last……detail…. has been calculated and thought out, allowing for the best chance of having a remarkable getaway! Sometimes, for me, the planning and researching for the trip can be almost as much fun as the trip itself, not quite, but almost! Admittedly, I do have a bit of apprehension prior to leaving, especially if we are flying to our vacation spot. Making sure we have appropriate identification, arriving on time at the gate, and finally landing safely at our destination. Still, having that plan in place before leaving provides me with a sense of security, minimizing any unforeseen circumstances that could put a significant damper on our much-needed downtime. Can the unexpected happen? Of course! The flight can be delayed or cancelled. Maybe the luggage doesn't arrive along with us to our vacation spot, but when you make proactive provisions, the opportunities for the unexpected can at the very least be minimized. Planning is the dough that holds the whole process together and creates a unique environment for success while minimizing issues that may lead to reactive decisions.

WHAT'S EATING YOU?

So, we are finally here! "Please secure your trays, put your seat in an upright position, and prepare for a smooth landing. My friends, we have reached the PREP FOR IT plan!" If you are a type A personality like me, it took everything inside of you not to skip through the first 7 chapters so you could get on with it already! As tempting as that might be, if you haven't gone through those chapters and done some soul searching, then this chapter is just instructions, not a game changer or a revelation. What is extremely important to grasp here, is no matter what eating plan works best for you (Clean eating plans, a point system, high fat/low carb, etc., etc.) without good preparation and a successful plan in place, it will only provide a temporary fix to a lifelong problem. The PREP FOR IT steps provide an opportunity to work through your specific issues and emotional roadblocks that cause you to become an emotional eater. The plan itself is formulated and implemented to create the vehicle to get you to the desired destination. When you invest just a few moments to sit down and formulate your strategy, i.e. the means by which you will execute your weight loss or wellness process, it will certainly give you the greatest chance for success. In addition, it will allow you to identify the emotional triggers that had the biggest impact on your fitness journey up to this point. Again, individualizing the plan for your specific goals will create the greatest chance for success. So how do we get there?

Individualize the Plan

Put your name on it! Own it! Make it all about you! You get the point. Everyone has something different they want to accomplish, different amounts of weight to lose, a different purpose or trigger that got them to this point, or even a wish or desire for your wellness and weight loss that you have kept locked up inside, never considering it could actually become reality. The purpose of the PREP FOR IT starter program, is to equip the reader or student with the necessary tools to ignite a change in your life. This will be the beginning of long-term success. Providing you with an easy, but thorough blueprint for your initial PREP FOR IT plan, creates an environment for you to start experiencing some wellness and weight loss successes!

You know, the best example I have for this is High School. Yep, we are going back to school, in more ways than one! In High School everyone took similar classes within the 4-year curriculum to get a high school diploma, and then inevitably moved on to college or a technical school based their chosen career path. What is so interesting to me, is that high school essentially taught the same lessons to all students. There were a few changes based on your desired career, destination. Nonetheless, the basics were taught to everyone. This holds true whether you were going to become a doctor or even an engineer. So how are the same programs that seem to be cookie cut, able to provide each individual exactly what he or she may need to succeed in their particular career choice? Here is the key...it's not the courses or classes, it's the individual's desired outcome and goals that are established before going into that class that provide a level of individuality. A great example, is when several people take biology. I always had a desire to become a medical professional, whether it was a doctor or a nurse, so when I took biology, I was stoked! Dissect a frog? Ah, yeah! More than likely, I looked at it a lot differently than someone who might be considering accounting as their career. Same classes, different goals. So, the outcome of what was learned was diverse, but effective. The aspiring accountant may have been indifferent to the class, just ensuring the box was checked off; whereas I relished each and every moment of the course. Same course, different aspirations. That is where PREP FOR IT academy comes into play. You may like whole/clean eating plans (paleo on caffeine!) or maybe you are an accountant and point counting sounds like the best recreational activity ever! Regardless of the eating plan, the premise behind what got you here and how you intend to remedy this will be somewhat the same. You can also follow the recipes we have made available in the resource chapter for meal options that follow a clean type of eating plan.

The point is, without a game plan, a desired outcome, and addressing the reason you landed here in the first place, you may be settling for short term wins without long-term successes. Don't get me wrong, I think there are some terrific eating plans out there. They provide great opportunities for weight loss, but again, we want you to identify the culprit that got you here. This way you, my friend, can finally say Arrivederci to that mulberry bush you have been circling for decades. You can use this plan to formulate and customize your game plan while using a popular or trendy eating plan based on food choices and other preferences. What makes that plan different for you is your effort. Delve into what brought you to this point and how to fix the things that could sabotage you along the way. Maybe mac and cheese are your nemesis. Or maybe it's the miniature peanut butter cups that keep you locked and loaded for the day. These are the areas we need to plan for to ensure your greatest success. Taking this step-by-step can help you formulate a plan that fits your needs, so sticking with this would be far easier than let's say, parallel parking downtown... in rush hour!

First things first: how much weight do you want to lose? It seems like a simple question, but most people will answer by saying, "A lot," or "50 pounds." Even if this is correct, how much weight do you want to lose right NOW? Consider short wins that will drive a positive momentum for an even greater reward. I would like to lose a pound a week Kelly. Great! Then exactly one year from now you would have lost 52 pounds. That was by simply making a few changes, consistently along the way. It was not an extreme assault on your daily routine that makes you feel deprived and frustrated. Implementing small goals will give you the taste of success you crave to bring on the even bigger wins.

The BMI (Body Mass Index) chart found in the supplemental workbook, will establish your ideal weight and help you formulate a weight loss goal. Body Mass Index is simply how much you weigh based on your height, to establish an ideal weight for you. There is a misconception that taller people should weigh more, and although there is some truth to this, that can be misleading and frankly, dangerous! The reality is that taller individuals just have more surface area to hide the weight better, but it's still there, believe me! Big point to realize is that the chart may say that based on your height and weight of 135 pounds, you are at a healthy weight. However, at 140 pounds you feel healthier and your clothes fit amazing, then 140 should be your goal. The BMI chart is just a guideline. It's not an absolute, but it does help you understand what would be considered the healthiest weight for you.

When I played college volleyball for a few years, I took time in the off season to lift weights and work out to improve my stamina and strength for the next season. We were fortunate to have the football strength and conditioning coach working with us, and he was so impressed and taken back that I could actually put a few plates on the bar before bench pressing! Ah the good ole days! I am digressing, but to make a valid point about weight, during my collegiate career, I was bench pressing my weight (which at the time was 135 pounds). That was an extremely big deal from both the perspective of upper-body strength and the fact that I was a female reaching this goal. I was in a size 5, and my fat ratio was below 15%. Now fast forward to 2 children and less time to dedicate to weight lifting with cardio workouts. I had stabilized at 135 pounds, but I was flirting with a size 8. My point is that I looked completely different at the same weight based on my current fitness level. Using the BMI will provide you a range but not an absolute to live within. When I discuss this with patients at our office, I try to use the example of 5 pounds of lead and 5 pounds of feathers in a bag. The lead would require a very small bag to hold the lead brick, but on the contrary, the feathers would need a much larger sack. Both are 5 pounds, but the density of the lead, takes up less room, therefore appears smaller and yes, even lighter. If you start becoming extremely active, then focusing on the weight may not provide all of the big wins you are desiring to see on the scale. Find the weight that makes you FEEL the healthiest and happiest. More importantly, find the weight that you are able to sustain long-term, and plan to take up residence there for a while!

Using the BMI scale is pretty easy, but for teaching purposes, we will use the following example. If you are 5'6" and you are 180 pounds then your BMI would be approximately 28-29. Now, this is not considered Obese, which the Obesity Medicine Association defines obesity as a BMI of 30 or greater, but it is considered overweight. According to the chart, if you could lose 25-30 pounds, then that would bring you into a normal BMI. Again, choosing your ideal weight will weigh heavily on what type of physical shape you plan to reach, as well as WHERE do you feel the absolute best? Going back to those impressionable years in high school, I had some pretty cool friends who I had the benefit of spending time with. They were fun, smart, and oh, all of them looked like little dress-up dolls. Petite frames and quite a bit shorter than I was. I felt like the Amazon in the room! I was definitely taller, and I don't ever think I was ever in a size zero (or for that matter a size 2). I looked like the odd man out! I had to realize that I was never going to LOOK like them or be their size without resembling a runway model on a 90-day hunger strike! I was thin and very physically fit, just not petite and tiny, and there really is, excuse the pun, a big difference! Find your happy weight, what makes you excited to get dressed and gives you a feeling of confidence when you walk out the door. Let that become the goal. It can always be re-evaluated when the time is right.

Once you have established your BMI, the next step is to determine in what time frame you would like to lose the weight. Remember, diets that tout you can lose 30 pounds in 30 days are probably diets that are pushing for the short-term goal and are likely not realistic. Many of these fad diets fail to help the participant identify the factors that catalyzed emotional eating causing most to fall short of achieving long term weight loss and the overall wellness. There are many amazing apps on smart phones now that provide a walk-through process to establish your daily caloric intake. They take your present weight and height (they then know your BMI), the time frame you are desiring for the weight loss, and based on your activity level, they establish a daily caloric intake for you. The apps are free with advertisements, but if you wanted to do some math on your own (Why?) then we provide the formula to walk through this process. According to the Journal of Strength and Conditioning Research, after conducting research comparing different BMI formulations, the Harris-Benedict Equation provides an overall easier method for calculation. Based on your specific needs, it will provide a well-proven estimation of your daily caloric needs.

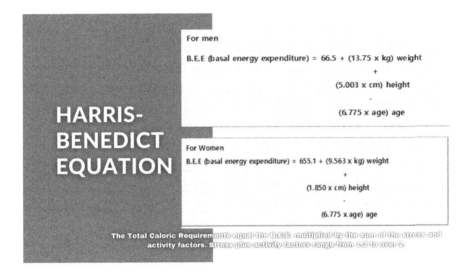

HARRIS-BENEDICT EQUATION

For men

B.E.E (basal energy expenditure) = 66.5 + (13.75 x kg) weight
+
(5.003 x cm) height
−
(6.775 x age) age

For Women

B.E.E (basal energy expenditure) = 655.1 + (9.563 x kg) weight
+
(1.850 x cm) height
−
(6.775 x age) age

The Total Caloric Requirements equal the B.E.E. multiplied by the sum of the stress and activity factors. Stress plus activity factors range from 1.2 to over 2.

Again, why try and make a wheel when there are great steel-belted ones online; don't sweat the laborious stuff! Typically these apps, when all the data is input, will give you a daily caloric intake to use as a target. Just get the app. There are plenty out there and if you are anything like me, it needs to be quick and easy! So, since you have decided to go with an app, (insert wink here!) you have now established your daily caloric intake. This is determined by your time-frame, your BMI and, of course, your activity level. This part is a huge determining factor in what you get to enjoy through the course of the day. It astounds me when I review this with patients in the office. When asked about exercise, it is either their version of what a silent movie would sound like, or they go on to tell me that their job is very active and they burn significant calories just making the Benjamins every day! Really?! Well, if that is the case, then they would be lean, mean fighting machines, right? Even if you are on your feet all day walking from room to room seeing patients, up and down on a stool in the exam room (yes, this is me), it is only considered lightly active. Why? Unless your job entails running from something at a pretty fast pace (zookeeper in a lion's den), or you sustain your heart rate at about 120 beats per minute for at least 20 minutes a day (aerobics instructor), then you, my friend, are just lightly active. Kelly, I lift boxes all day long, great! Still lightly active. Kelly, I am a personal shopper for online grocery ordering. Still…lightly active. Many individuals have a tendency to underestimate their caloric intake but often overestimating their activity level. This is likely why we find ourselves dealing with a higher BMI and sticking to the accessory aisle of the department stores. The best advice I can give you here is this. If you eat more than you put out in energy, you will inevitably gain weight. Period. You have to be able to find that daily caloric intake which allows you to feel satiated, like you are not missing a thing, all while still having the ability to see a decrease on the scale.

Three Important Questions

We will get into the meat of planning in just one moment, but it is imperative at least weekly to ask yourself those 3 simple questions we referred to earlier. First, "Am I eating the right foods every day and avoiding the wrong foods (this includes alcohol)?" Secondly, "Am I eating the right number of calories every day? Not too many, where I stand to gain weight if not monitored and not less than 800 calories a day, where the body feels it is in starvation mode and will slow the metabolism down for survival?" Finally, "Am I exercising on a regular basis?" Again, you don't need to be a tri-athlete, but you need to have some form of cardio in your routine at least 2 to 3 times weekly. If the answer to any of these questions is no, then you must focus on the area that is insufficient to ensure that you are not sabotaging your forward progress.

I had a patient in the clinic some time ago who was distraught. She was complaining about her inability to lose 10 pounds despite EVERY effort and requested an appetite suppressant.

"Uh, no, I am not giving you a stimulant for you to get quick, empty results only to stop the medication in 3 months and gain that weight and a few extra hitch-hikers along the way!" So, I asked her the 3 glass-check questions. She admitted that she wasn't eating the wrong foods, but she was drinking 2 glasses of wine every night. I know, in the South, that can sound like par for the course, but for her, it was creating a negative impact in her life. So, we talked about the wine intake. It is similar to drinking a liquid snicker bar, and it could be the source of her issues. When we discussed this a little further, I asked when did she begin drinking 2 glasses of wine a night. She responded, approximately 18 months ago. I then asked, (this is very, very important) "What happened 18 months ago? Was there anything significant that may have occurred around that time?"

She looked stunned, really stunned, but I could see this lightbulb go off above her head and she mumbled, "Our house flooded, and we lost everything and had to gut our home." Hmmm? This sounds like a big event that may have caused the emotional monster to take a walk on the wild side and wreak havoc in her life for the past 18 months. It was her coping mechanism during such a stressful and devastating time. She became an emotional drinker (not eater) but it affected her the same, exact way! Remember a calorie, is a calorie, is a calorie. Whether it is a bowl of mac and cheese, a margherita, or a bit of mint chocolate chip ice cream, it can affect us all the same way. The funny thing about this encounter is after we identified the catalyst, (what created the change and allowed her to fuel her emotions with food or in this case, alcohol) she never asked me for the medications again. She realized that the power to make the change and control the emotional monster was within her the entire time. She just didn't realize it. Really making a concerted effort to find out if there is a culprit and what you can do to minimize its control in your life truly becomes life-changing. It can forever alter the course of your wellness and weight loss journey in a positive way. There are additional things we need to discuss to facilitate keeping the emotional monster locked up and controlled.

The Choice is Yours

When selecting a diet to assist you with your weight loss and wellness goals, you need to research what is feasible, and still allows you to achieve long-term success. As you choose an eating plan, consider what will work best for your taste preferences, schedule, and financial capabilities. It is crucial to understand the types of calories the plan allows, having a basic knowledge of the different food groups, and weighing the pro's and con's, to determine the best plan for your health and lifestyle. Every eating plan will have a specific formulation that will allow the participant to achieve maximum results. However, they are essentially broken down into 3 caloric groups: proteins, carbohydrates, and fats. According to the United States Department of Health, these are further broken down into 5 major food groups: Breads/cereals/grains, fruits, vegetables and legumes, milk/cheese/yogurt, and lean meats (chicken, fish, beef, eggs and nuts). While most diets focus on limiting the caloric intake to ensure that you are expending more calories than you are ultimately consuming, many of the newer diets on the market have focused on certain combinations of these caloric or food groups. The high protein/low carbohydrate plans, which have recently garnered much attention, attempt to restrict the carbohydrate calories that require less thermal energy to burn. When this occurs, it essentially forces your body to produce its own glucose mainly through the liver to help sustain your energy through the course of the day. When this happens, you are able to use the protein and fat supplies stored in the body to obtain the materials to produce this energy. When caloric limitations are set, weight loss will inevitably occur because the energy will need to come from somewhere. If you are anything like me, you may have a little fat to spare! We have placed a food group list, along with the calories per serving, in the supplemental workbook to provide an easy reference to you when you are looking for low carbohydrate options. We purposely did not include calories/serving for PREP FOR IT recipes because I truly believe that portion control, healthy eating, and understanding that eating is a function takes the mathematical stress out of weight loss and overall wellness.

Again, there are plenty of amazing eating plans out there right now that incorporate healthy, gluten-free or grain-free options, allowing your body to run on premium fuel. My personal preference lies somewhere between a modified paleo-type, clean eating plan. I do think that if you are trying to lose weight and you are not seeing expected results with the effort you are putting into the plan, then you need to consider shaking things up. These two particular plans remind me a lot of a computer that goes awry. When your computer does starts stalling, maybe acting a little weird or even freezes up altogether, what do you typically do to attempt to get it working again? You reboot it! Clean eating plans allow you to go back to whole foods, no artificial anything, as many whole ingredients as possible and removing possible triggers such as dairy (milk proteins), and even grains for at least 1 month. They help to reboot your internal computer so that it can work at its peak performance. We are not set on one particular eating plan, just the steps you take to address what got you here in the first place. I believe that when you go through the PREP FOR IT process, acknowledge what got you to this point, and make the necessary changes to keep the emotional monster in check, you will see success on any eating plan that works well for you.

I also think it is important when you begin this journey to make an appointment with your provider to ensure you are not going to be fighting an uphill battle. Many times, we see patients who are trying very hard to achieve weight loss and overall wellness, yet they are at a firm standstill, not even a subtle budge on the ole scale. They will often come into the office very frustrated and disenchanted and may even be on the verge of giving up. There are blood tests that can be drawn, to see if there are certain medical conditions that could be hindering their progress. For example, if you have a Vitamin D deficiency, thyroid dysfunction or a metabolic disorder you could follow a strict eating plan to a tee for the entire month, and then step onto the scale only to find that you have not seen an ounce of weight loss. Talk about discouraging. Simply because you are deficient in a much-needed vitamin or hormone for normal bodily functions to occur. Your provider can review any signs and symptoms you are having and offer some medical testing, specific to you, that could potentially identify any culprits before you begin this journey of a lifetime.

Must Haves

So, no matter what diet or eating plan you choose to assist you on this journey, there are a few must-haves in your plan that are non-negotiables in order to obtain optimum success. Proactive planning is a must to ensure less reactive choices that become bad habits. We talked about this several chapters back, but it is extremely important for you to understand this concept. What you think about before you encounter an issue or extreme change in emotion will weigh heavily on what you will actually do when the time comes… and it will. Remember, we need to realize the emotional monster is always ready and waiting in the wings to wreak havoc on our overall wellness and weight loss goals. We just need to be able to give him a good glass check (hockey term) when we inevitably have to deal with an extreme emotion during the course of our day.

Next, food prepping for the week is essential. Is it fun? Sometimes it is lots of fun. Sometimes it feels like any other chore that you need to do over the course of the weekend. Laundry done, check. House cleaned, check. Food prepped for the week, check. Once you realize how important prepping is and how easy it will make the rest of the week, getting on board becomes far easier. I like to think of this a bit like an investment. I am putting in the time on a Saturday or Sunday so that I don't have to do squat the rest of the week. Well, when you say it like that Kelly, let's do this! Right!?! Some even opt to make enough for a few weeks and freeze what they are able to in order to become even more efficient, but if you are like me, once I freeze something, it goes into the great frozen abyss never to be seen again! Food prep does take a significant amount of discipline, time, and effort. However, when you complete the task and take a peek into your fridge at all of the options that lie before you, it is such a feeling of accomplishment and believe it or not, a level of peace and calmness will often set in, fending off the potential attacks planned by the emotional monster. "An ounce of prevention is worth a pound of cure." Keep in mind, that the planning and prepping you do during your valuable free time will allow you the needed restorative time during the week. This should be more than enough motivation to stick with the program and keep up the good work! You will seriously thank me later, especially during the hectic weekdays when you open the fridge door and can almost hear the sound of a church choir singing aaa....ahhhhhh!!!!

Food prepping is not a new concept; in fact, many little creatures living in the wild are professionals at food prepping. It's what they do. It is a direct function for survival to meet the needs when the time is right. It's not to celebrate hump day, or National Donut Day, or Johnny's quiz score for the week. We need to glean something from our furry rodent friends and what they are accomplishing. Food prepping needs to become part of your life-style, part of your routine, and once you can get into a flow, it becomes a major contributor to your long-term success with wellness and weight loss. There are a few things that are essential to your success with food prep. If your desire is for weight loss, we suggest making sure that you are using all organic products and non-GMO (genetically modified) where possible.

Organic products are meats and produce that have been grown or raised in a natural surrounding with no chemicals, or hormone exposure. Studies suggest that the chemicals and hormones that food has been exposed to have been linked to autoimmune disorders, chronic stomach and bowel issues and may even be associated with some cancers. GMO (genetically modified organism) is simply any organism whose genetic material or makeup has been altered using genetic engineering techniques. Originally, this genetic modification was intended to enhance the virility and resistance of seeds and plants. This, in turn, would produce better, larger produce that could resist the threats of pests and damaging growth. The intent was to make the organism (seed or plant) stronger by allowing it to withstand exposure to pests, extreme weather, and soil conditions. We are beginning to realize that we really are what we eat. Research has identified that long-term exposure to these GMO products is increasing many chronic health issues in humans. Our bodies were not made to tolerate the harsh chemicals and changes from these products. In addition, if you are really trying to reboot your body, I would further suggest (for at least an initial period of one to two months) removing any milk or dairy products, grains or legumes, and refined starches/carbohydrates.

What are carbs Kelly? Basically, carbohydrates are rice, potatoes, bread/flour products, sweets-essentially all of the foods that are yummy, yummy, for your tummy! These are the foods that may have "comforted" you in the past. Side note, think about it, people will often refer to certain meals as their comfort food (mac and cheese, mashed potatoes, potato chips, cheesecake lol) and many of the foods that we associate with making us "feel" better are actually carbohydrates that are full of empty calories and will often leave us feeling horrible and worse...wanting for more! So much hate?!

To successfully food prep, we recommend establishing menus for the week ahead of time to give you ample time to go grocery shopping and obtain necessary seasonings and such. Don't tell me you don't have time to grocery shop, my friend. Many large supermarkets now shop for you and even deliver. Just remember, excuses (cough, cough! Rationalization) will get you no further than you already are. Just go ahead and get rid of them so you can get on with a better, healthier you! You need to become very methodical with prepping. Put your menu together, make the grocery list, shop, and prep. Put your menu together, make the grocery list, shop, and prep. You get the point. Make it a habit just like any other chore that you would get done through the course of your week. We have put together a 6-week food prep starter course that gives the reader step-by-step instructions to go from soup to nuts with food prepping, and it takes a lot of the guesswork out of prepping. We have put together 30 amazing entrees and over 20 different side dishes (the recipes are also located in the resource chapter of this book) along with copies of the recipes and the grocery lists that can be printed for each week. The six-week course covers 5 lunches and dinners through the week with 2 days of planning that you can cater specifically to what you have a desire to eat or maybe even crave. Again, we realize that everyone has different levels of proficiency when it comes to food preparation, following recipes, and feeling comfortable in the kitchen. If you are a novice, please do not let food prep intimidate you. Start small and simple. The easy-to-make meals can provide you with quick wins and then as you gain confidence, start delving into some of the more complex recipes. On a follow up visit with a patient, she admitted that roasted vegetables had amazing flavor, and she couldn't believe how easy they were to prepare. YOU CAN DO THIS!

Breakfast and Snacks

What about breakfast and snacks Kelly? Great question. There are some menus provided in the supplemental workbook, but let me say this about breakfast or any meal for that matter. Food is a function, plain and simple. Yes, you will have opportunities to have a celebratory meal, but every meal is not an occasion; it is just another task in your daily routine. Become habitual in your breakfast and snack choices. Why? When these meals become habitual routines, then it removes the highs and emotional lows that you can have that may be associated with the meal. I am extremely habitual with my breakfast and snacks. On any given morning, my breakfast will consist of several different combinations that will look something like this: a boiled egg and

2 pieces of organic breakfast sausage, almond yogurt with grain-free granola (this also can double as a snack which is great), an apple and a boiled egg, an apple and breakfast sausage, an egg and 2 small pieces of uncured bacon, or an apple with uncured breakfast sausage. It's like playing Tetris with your food! How many different combinations can I put together with these 3 or 4 items? It is just a morning task, which allows me to remove the emotional tie to this particular meal. Do I love a great breakfast? Uh, yeah! It is absolutely my favorite of all the meals. There are times when I will make breakfast a special occasion. It may be a weekend outing with my husband to kick-start the weekend and my food prepping, or when my daughter and her family are in for a weekend visit. Pick your battles, and make them count. Believe it or not, when you start to implement this mind-set, you really start to see those special meals for what they are and enjoy not just the food, but you fully engage and enjoy everything about it. Now, I want to mention something here. Breakfast doesn't need to be bland to be functional. We have some great recipes in the supplemental workbook for some egg muffin frittatas, pumpkin pancakes and even muffins in a mug! These recipes provide you with high protein, low carbohydrate meal options that will help you to kick-start your day the right way, all while tasting great!

Snacks are no different. When you look in my purse, it will often resemble a healthy version of the nearest convenience store. You may find a bag of mixed nuts, beef jerky, possibly an apple, protein chips, or even a protein bar. Before I walk out of the door on any given day, I take a few minutes to actually run through, in my mind, what my day may look like and make all of the necessary preparations. Does this seem like overkill? At first, it might. However, when you get into a rhythm, it is no different than making your coffee first thing in the morning or brushing your teeth before you walk out the door. It's just another part of my morning routine. Remember that by making these plans ahead of time, you are creating an environment that minimizes reactive choices which can lead you down that dark path to the Specialty coffee line for a vanilla cream Frappe with white chocolate curls! I recommend not only preparing for your week at work or school, but also, I strongly urge you to continue to implement this practice on the weekends as well. Truly, you are more apt to slip up when you are not in a typical daily routine, and if you are anything like me, weekends usually resemble the end of the movie Grease when everyone ran out of the school at the end of the year screaming and waving their hands in the air!

Hopefully you have begun to get a clearer picture of what food prepping will look like in your home. Get pumped to start implementing some proactive planning in your life that will reduce those reactive choices that have been wreaking havoc for so long! This part is really exciting! It's kind of like getting a present that you had been wanting and are finally getting that chance to start using it. Okay, maybe it's not quite like that, but if you are anything like me, it is exciting to begin with a fresh slate, envisioning what the end result will look and feel like.

If you have decided to use the 6-week PREP FOR IT starter course, then you can simply follow along with the recipes, grocery lists and weekly play-by-play handout that are provided for each week in the series. Our goal was to remove the stress of planning which would allow you the time needed to establish great proactive habits. If you want to customize a plan for you, simply go through the supplemental workbook of the book and start planning what your meals for lunch and dinner will look like for the week first. Get a prep notebook and write out what you want to eat for the week which includes your entrees and sides. One thing I strongly recommend is providing a broad variety of foods each week so that you don't find yourself in chicken or fish burnout, which can be detrimental to avoid derailment as your wellness train is just picking up speed; seriously this can happen and when it does, it's hard to snap out of it! Once you have established the menu for the week, simply go through each recipe and put together a grocery list. This is imperative, my friends! Why? What's the big deal? Remember, your goal is to be proactive here, and one thing I know is when you step into a grocery store, the possibility for you to trip, slip, or simply drive off the deep end by putting stuff in that buggy of yours that doesn't need to be there is very probable. So, get the grocery list together, stuff it in your purse or wallet, and put on a dab of determination before you head out the door to make this food prep thing happen!

There are a few suggestions that I want to offer here in particular. If you can, make shopping for your food items a function too; it does help to minimize the reactive choices that happen on your way to check-out. Try to stay to the outside areas of the grocery first. What is the deal Kelly?!? Grocers are in the business to make money, not necessarily to make you healthy, so many items that are not good for you, that are convenient, in cardboard boxes just waiting for you to add water, mix and enjoy, are typically found either in the middle or end sections of the grocery store aisles. Typically, the dairy, produce, and meats are on the outer edges of the grocery and that is where you really need to focus most of your energy. If you don't have 3 hours to set aside to get the food prep done for the week, there are a few things that can help to ease this burden as well. Many of the grocery stores realize that people are trying to eat healthier and eat more whole and organic food options, so they actually are trying to provide convenient options for you when it comes to even food-prepping. They may have zucchini already noodled, cauliflower already riced in the frozen or fresh food sections; they may even have some of the ingredients in one container where you simply take the cover off, place it in a heated oven and let her go! If you are making certain dishes such as the pecan crusted trout, getting finely chopped pecans instead of whole pecans does alleviate a couple of steps in the process. Certainly, these are all great options if you know that you can't spend very long getting the entrees and sides together, but you will pay to play, so be prepared! Most often the grocer will charge you more for the cubed butternut squash, pound for pound than the whole squash that you will need to peel and cube at home. Is this cheating? Absolutely not! Do what will work best for you in the long run. Just realize that it may cost a little more on the front end to help you with the prepping on the back end. We want to create positive momentum that over time will lead to long-term results, so anything that allows you to have sticking power is A-Okay in my book!

It isn't necessary to assign certain foods for a particular day of the week, unless you enjoy the overwhelming control that it gives you. I prefer to make all of the entrees and sides. then place them in larger containers so that from day to day, it allows me to choose the lunch and dinner for the day. This is actually a really fun part for my husband and I. When we get home in the evening, he may say he wants to eat the chicken wings and a sweet potato and I may have been waiting all day to sink my teeth into the barbacoa beef (yes, it's that off the hook!). One of the great parts about prepping for the week, is it allows for deviations to the original plan without compromising the ultimate goal. Having the ability to choose what meal you will eat and when, all while still seeing great results can truly become a motivator in and of itself.

Drop and Give Me 20!

We will talk briefly about the next topic of discussion because, yes, my friends, we have a whole chapter devoted to the topic of exercise. Listen, I get it. You don't want to be married to the gym, you want to have firm legs and feel healthy, but spending hours upon hours in classes or on the gym floor isn't what you really had in mind. I totally understand. I strongly recommend for the first 2 to 3 months minimizing your exercise to only mild-moderate cardio workouts to keep the metabolism up. I know what you are probably thinking, "Yes!! Finally, no exercise to reach the end goal!" Nah, that is not what I said. What I want you to focus on initially is addressing the emotional monster, proactively planning your meals and making healthier choices, all while starting to increase your daily activity level. The reason for this is I want you to obtain the benefits of the initial cardio workouts, but if one of your desired outcomes is to lose inches, initially that may not happen with strenuous exercise, and this could have the potential of becoming very discouraging. Remember, we want those quick wins that will help you to gain the momentum you need to conquer the next level with a greater chance for success.

Once I had been prepping for several months, I started to get a feeling that I needed to up my game when it came to my physical activity. Yes, I worked in the yard and even did an occasional stent on the treadmill upstairs, but I felt the need to make some greater changes in this particular area. I joined a group fitness class that is very structured and extremely challenging. Let's put it this way. It's the closest thing to legalized torture, at least from my perspective, and I actually pay them to torture me! I go to the one-hour class about 2 days a week, and then try to get in another day of some moderate cardio as well. This has been a game changer for my energy level, stamina, and physical appearance. One thing to note here: when you start to gear up your metabolism, your appetite is not too far behind. I noticed that I was hungrier after exercising, and if you are not careful at this point, Rationalization will make its way back into your life by simply convincing you that since you have increased your physical activity, then those cookies in the break room are totally ok, and that king cake? Why sure! Don't fall for it! You worked very hard to get to this point, not to allow any part of emotional eating to find its way back into your life. Again, we will talk more on this subject in the next chapter, but just start somewhere and before you know it, you are there!

Glass Check It!

So, you have established what your weight loss and wellness goals are at this point and started the PREP FOR IT 6-week course. That's incredible! Make sure to look for the positives when making these changes to your life and eating habits, as this is crucial in providing a means of forward momentum. With that said, it is imperative that weekly you do what I like to call glass-checking. In hockey, a player can slam the opponent onto the glass, and to me, this is the epitome of the wake-up call. Every week, we should be taking a good, hard look at our progress. Celebrate the wins, identify the opportunities, and revisit our PREP FOR IT steps, if necessary, to ensure that we are continuing to make forward progress. Why is this so important? I'll tell you why, because life happens whether you have implemented new strategies or not. It will come at you, barrels locked, loaded, and ready to go! You will get flat tires, have issues at work or with a customer, miss out on the promotion, break-up with a boyfriend, and even worse, maybe experience a tragic event. The whole mind-set here is to establish proactive plans that reduce the reactive choices; it doesn't get rid of the events that can unfortunately lead to these decisions. When faced with the inevitable issues of the week, maybe you rationalized a particular food or meal choice and need to just go back through that process and what it means to remove Rationalization from the equation and what that would look like for future food choices. Possibly, your expectations about the progress you intended to make this week was skewed and may need a bit of revision to become more realistic, allowing you to establish the positive momentum that you need through the process. Maybe through the course of 6 to 8 weeks you have found yourself trying a few shortcuts related to snack planning and wandered away from the healthy options that have worked well as a function up to this point in your journey. Is it possible that you have prepped less this week as a result of a busy schedule or an unforeseen circumstance that developed.

    We know that life will have its Ups and yes, inevitably its Downs and we need to make sure at the very least that we are checking the engine weekly to ensure all is working well and nothing is in need of an overhaul! Evaluate the meals. What did you love? What was good but not necessarily your favorite? Start documenting this to help you with your future meal plans. Prep, Eat, Evaluate, Repeat. Prep, Eat, Evaluate, Repeat. It's that simple. When you can become methodical in your weekly plan and goals, you will curtail the emotional monster's ability to wreak havoc and finally take that much needed control over your life!

CHAPTER 9

Slips, Trips, and Pitfalls

Many times, as you begin something new, or incorporate a new process into your life, you can be taken back and entrapped by the pitfalls that may lie inconspicuously in your path. These are the unknown issues that have not been taken into account or may have been concealed from you as you embarked on this new journey. The same is true about the actual pitfall traps used to ensnare wild animals or those unknowing beasts that fall unaware into the entrenchment concealed in ground cover. Both are moving forward to a specific destination. The animal will find himself wrapped up and entangled in the pit awaiting its predator. Likewise, you have been making incredible headway in this weight loss and wellness journey only to find yourself in a little bit of a tailspin with the emotional monster hot on your trail. The unforeseen issues don't occur because of a lack of planning or gained insight into the change you have elicited. They can happen despite even the best laid plans.

Realizing that slip-ups and pitfalls are a part of life will contribute significantly to your outlook and your ultimate success with this program. In layman's terms, stuff happens, so be prepared! We touched on this briefly in the last chapter, but I wanted to take a few minutes to not only cheer you on, but also to prepare you for what lies ahead. Do you think for one minute that the emotional monster that has been having a hay-day in your life is just simply going to bow out and exit curtain left? No, indeed! I can make one promise here. At least for the first few weeks, when you start to incorporate the PREP FOR IT acronyms in your life and proactively plan out your meals, you my friend, will be miserable! Great Kelly! You are doing an awesome job selling this concept!

Thanks for the pep talk, Kelly! (insert image of me sarcastically, giving you a double thumbs up!) Look, anything of value or worth doesn't just happen because we thought it up or wrote it down on a piece of paper. No, no. When you want to change the direction of the Titanic, you need to be prepared to hit a few icebergs. Maybe not the best example as the plight of this ship was dismal. Nonetheless, you need to be prepared for what lies ahead and don't always make decisions based on what you may see just above the surface.

Often times, you will meet individuals who reveal amazing transformations. They have lost over 100 pounds in a year. Maybe they have completed a triathlon after strenuous training and conditioning, or maybe you have run into an individual who had an addictive disorder, and they have been drug or alcohol free for over 3 years. What do all of these individuals have in common? At some point, they experienced the Aha moment, took control of the situation in their lives, and reached the goal that they had set for themselves. You may also run into individuals who reach many of the same feats as these have and yet, within just a few years, they have either regained the weight, or couldn't trot to the front door, let alone train for a marathon. You think to yourself, "What in the world happened?" To the outsider, it can seem like they lost some of their passion or desire to stick with the goal, but for these individuals, it started with a slip-up that turned into another slip-up that turned into being off the wagon (just a little), to finally succumbing to the easier, less challenging option of letting go. Letting go doesn't start with the first, second, or for that matter the 10th slip-up. It happens when someone loses the focus of the goal that they originally had in mind, and over time, it just becomes easier to stop putting in the extra effort. Additionally, when we become so focused on a specific goal and not the process and life-style change at hand, we could be setting ourselves up for failure before we even leave the dock.

I have many patients with BMIs well over 50 who have needed to lose substantial amounts of weight. They've tried multiple diet attempts, eating plans, medications, and even therapies to no avail. Many turned to weight loss surgery as a means of catalyzing a rapid weight loss, to gain the much-needed traction, and SEE the results that they needed. I have been fortunate to work with many of them through the entire transformation, immediately after surgery, then months after, when the weight was melting off. I could see their confidence rise. They glowed! It was truly incredible to witness. I remember having conversations with some of them about their plans for maintaining the loss after they reached their desired goals. Many had amazing plans in place. Others stated that they would just "eat healthier." Sadly, several of my patients, over the course of a few years, gained most, if not all of the weight back. They would show up at the clinic discouraged, frustrated, and sometimes heavier than when they first began their journeys.

How, did this happen?? I can only use experience here to shed a little light onto this particular issue. When you start on the journey, there is more structure. You are almost obsessive/compulsive when it comes to the planning and execution. Why? Because when you have the Aha moment that we mentioned earlier and you decide enough is enough, then you will do anything and everything you can to establish a platform for success. If the program or eating plan tells you to do A and B, and it will result in C, my guess is that you will be "all onboard" to do A and B exactly like they are recommending to ensure you see the expected results of C (Finally!! I got to use something from my logic class in college!) Then as you start to see the initial results, it can become an incredible motivator and fuels the fire to implement additional strategies for results. Don't get me wrong. The struggles are very real, and they start with the first day of change, but the resolve you feel when you start the plan drives the ship past the initial obstacles to help achieve some smooth sailing along the way. However, as we alluded to earlier, stuff happens.

Let me further explain this concept. Imagine your weight loss and wellness goals like a car that has to get to the top of the mountain. The mountain itself can seem daunting, but at the bottom of this vast rock, you put the petal to the metal, and you floor it! You buy every single ingredient they tell you to get. In fact, you may have even had to travel far and wide to obtain them. You read the eating or diet plan numerous times until you can blurt out the premise and guidelines in your sleep. You are full steam ahead and even starting to see some progress. The mountain isn't so big. I got this! This isn't as hard as I thought it would be. You think this while still at the lower third of the mountain. Don't get me wrong. Having steam at the beginning of the journey is extremely important, but this is not a sprint. Remember, we are in a marathon for life. As you make your way up the mountain, or in this case, through the pant sizes, you get a certain degree of comfort and a feeling that the effort required is not as significant now as it may have been in the beginning. I like to refer to this as the, "I got this" mentality. It's the feeling you have that tells you it's not necessary to put the full effort into the program or strategies to see the needed results because you are making forward progress even with a few slip-ups. STOP! Here is where your buggy will lose some serious steam and fast! This is simple physics. If a vehicle is going up an incline, it takes power and force to create positive momentum. In order to get to the top of the mountain, the vehicle MUST continue to push at the same or even stronger pace, depending on the incline, to reach its destination. In the middle of this journey, any time the driver of the vehicle (that's you!) decides to put the car in neutral and coast the rest of the way, they will ultimately find themselves back at the starting point. In fact, if you lose the traction that you obtained initially up the steep incline, you can create just as much momentum going down the mountain and find yourself even further away from the starting point than when you initially began. In other words, not only do you gain the weight back, but you pick up a few hitch-hikers (pounds) on the way down!

 Weight loss and obtaining true wellness takes time. It takes a plan, and it takes a resolve within you to stay on the journey for the long haul, not just for a few months. So, when you start reaching some initial goals (going down a dress/pant size), or you are able to finally plank for 30 seconds, there is a slight change in the atmosphere that, frankly, can be deadly. There is an air or aura, sense of comfort, ease, and possibly even a bit of overconfidence. If this occurs, and for many it is inevitable, then you have a tendency to let your guard down and not focus on the basics. Just remember, "keep it simple sweetheart." This literally means don't overthink, complicate, or create obstacles unnecessarily. Stick to the basics, and you will never go wrong. It is when we start to gain confidence that we must hunker-down even more. Become more focused and determined to stay on the journey. It is for this reason that I strongly recommend not establishing a goal for a specific life event or activity (I am losing 30 pounds before my high school reunion; I am going down 3 pant sizes before my daughter's wedding). Achieving these goals are amazing, but should never be the primary reason for your desired weight loss or wellness. If you have decided to eat healthier and lose a little weight in the process, then start as soon as you have the equipment, resources and time.... just begin. Begin somewhere. Even with small changes, you would be astounded to see the progress you can make with consistent small choices over a long period of time. Look, if it is a Tuesday or even a Thursday, you have the same opportunity for success as those who started on New Year's Day. In fact, you may have a greater chance for success!

For some, you may need to write the plan for your fitness and weight loss and put them in places that are visible and allow them to act as daily reminders to stick with it, even when you may not be feeling it. Others may like visuals and post a picture of what they look like and a picture of what they want to achieve based on their overall desires. (Be realistic here, throw the runway model brochures out. We all know those girls eat 2 stalks of celery a day, please!) Maybe the picture is from the past when you were leading a more disciplined life and eating healthier. Maybe there is a particular outfit that you like or have that you would love to wear. Again, make sure that you are starting this journey for the right reasons because when you accomplish the specific goal you set out to achieve, many times it's like getting to a finish line, throwing the flag over your shoulders to take the victory laps, all while asking to have a cheeseburger. When this happens, it signifies the end of the race, a need to celebrate and let your guard down after all of those long months of training and healthy eating. That can be a major pitfall. We don't want to see you put a book end to this experience. We want this to be a life-long journey that brings you joy, happiness, and wellness. Reaching the specific goal creates a beginning and unfortunately, an end to what you are trying to reach. Of course, you don't want to be extremely vague with what you would like to accomplish either. You just don't want to pigeon hole yourself into a certain time frame. This can create unwanted stress, which can become another pitfall. Then guess who is knocking and wants to play for a bit! Referencing our previous analogy, our journey with long-term weight loss and wellness resembles a ride going up an escalator rather than a mountain climb. When climbing or racing up a mountain, you will eventually reach the peak, an end to the established goals that were set. Lifetime wellness and weight loss, like an escalator, requires a continued focus on the steps before you with a need to maintain the climb.

It's the Real Deal

What do you mean? Well, let's say you want to lose 30 pounds, but you set a goal that you want to lose half of this weight in the first month (not realistic). As you get closer to that deadline, if you are behind schedule, you're likely not close to reaching the first checkpoint. This can be very counterproductive to what you are trying to accomplish, with the potential to experience increased stress. If you are the emotional eater that I think you might be (based on your desire to read this book), then you have told the emotional monster, "Sure, let's go a few rounds with no gloves on, sounds awesome!?!" You are adding a factor that could actually make you more prone to slipping up and going southside for some cupcakes or muffins. You are trying to block him out, for that matter, starve him out! You want to create an ongoing atmosphere of proactivity and reduce any chances that may cause you to slip away. Go back to your basics. Be regimented with your meals and your snacks almost ad nauseam. Be realistic. Understand that if goals are not realistic, you may need to re-evaluate to create the best platform for your success in this journey.

Control the Fall

Plan for the slip-ups! What? In? The? World? Yes! Plan for them! Planning for the slip-ups can create opportunities for minimal damage through this process of change. For example, let's say you have a building that is beyond repair and needs to be demolished. The demo team will actually provide very calculated measures to ensure that the destruction of the building or implosion is calculated and controlled. The building is still going to fall out into millions of pieces, but by strategic planning, the crew provides an environment to reduce the aftershock or unexpected fall-outs. Now, let's make this relatable. Say you have an upcoming anniversary and your spouse has decided to surprise you with a dinner at one of the finest dining establishments in the South. By all means have a blast…. within reason. Look ahead at the upcoming train, I mean meal and see how you would like to handle the situation. Review the menu ahead of time and make a great choice now. I will eat the fish or chicken with the vegetables, so that I can have a couple of bites of the anniversary dessert they bring to the table. In that celebratory atmosphere, when you show up dressed to the nines and the waiter offers you the menu, block out the temptation to say, "Sure, I'll take a look! Why, yes, I'll have the pasta and shrimp dish with garlic mashed potatoes on the side, and absolutely bring us the dessert menu after the meal!" Having a few bites of the dessert is not going to be your downfall. It's when you go into a situation ill-prepared that will open up Pandora's cake box.

Breaking the Boredom Cycle

A common pitfall that many, many dieters and healthy eaters alike encounter is the sheer monotony of a healthy eating plan. Humans, notoriously are creatures of habit, but we do want the environment around us to change a little along the way. Many fad diets out there offer short-term results because many of the foods are repetitious in nature and you simply drink the same shake over and over and over again. Or you eat chicken and fish every day to the point you start noticing feathers and gills when you look in the mirror. Yes, even prepping can become a little boring. Yes, I said it! Remember our mission is to make your meals a function not an occasion, but it doesn't have to taste bland. You should never feel like you are missing out on anything while you are trying to achieve your set goals. The recipes we provided in the resource chapter are meant to create variety. We wanted to cover a broad span of food groups, ethnic variations, and introduce you to new vegetables and food combinations. Variety is the spice of life, and it absolutely can prevent boredom when you are trying to lose weight or obtain better health. Make it a mission to look for new takes on your old favorites. Scour the health food stores and groceries for new healthier snack options and push yourself to try new things. When we allow creativity to play a part in our plan, then we are more inclined to stay on board for the long ride.

Paint the Barn Door

A dear friend of mine, who was a local Obstetrician, had a saying he shared with me. I was trying to start my own OB home health company at the time, and as we were brainstorming and mulling over a few things, he said, "Kelly, you are just going to have to paint the barn door until the paint sticks." I have held onto that adage for over 30 years now, and it is more pertinent now than it was even back then. Essentially, to create permanent change in your wellness and weight loss journey, you need to put your hip boots on and be prepared to dig a deep and lasting foundation. One of the toughest pitfalls with weight loss occurs when someone is following all of the instructions EXACTLY like they are supposed to, following all of the rules and breaking none, only to find that they may have made little to no progress at the first checkpoint or weigh-in. This can be extremely frustrating for anyone! Realize there are several factors that may influence how quickly you are able to create positive momentum. Your age, activity level, and even metabolic disorders, such as thyroid disease or insulin resistance, can create a significant resistance at the onset of the journey. If you continue to make the small changes, consistently over time and stay focused and steadfast, you will eventually see a change. If you do follow a plan without any diversion, and you are still struggling with losing weight along the way, then seeing your provider may be necessary to ensure there are no other issues that are creating resistance. Again, one of the most common conditions that many individuals currently suffer with is Vitamin D deficiency. This has become a bigger issue with people trying to stay out of the sun and avoiding milk which has been fortified with Vitamin D. Without this particular Vitamin, your body will politely pull-over at a rest stop and stall your weight loss journey. You may consider seeing your provider and have a panel of bloodwork done prior to starting this journey to ensure there are no obstacles that may delay any positive momentum you will experience.

Modern demands require plans that push for microwave results, fast and easy. True long-term wellness and weight loss still requires a slow cooker process to achieve the goals. So, maybe you don't lose a pound a week, maybe you lose 1/2 pound a week; then in a year you still lost 26 pounds, and that is still something to celebrate! So, I implore you to paint the barn door 'til the paint sticks. Make each and every day count. Even the small changes that may seem insignificant: giving up sweet tea, (oh that girl did not just say that?!?) drinking more water, removing an unnecessary snack after work, walking briskly for 30 minutes, 3 times a week. Seriously, the list is endless, and the cool thing is you create your own course for success!

Get Over It Already!

We are all human and very fallible, so we need to understand that we will experience slip-ups. We will acquiesce and have a little bit of cookie cake for our co-worker's retirement party. I mean, come on Kelly, she is retiring! I know, I get it. Remember, I was in the same boat as you. Still, an ice-berg is an ice-berg is an iceberg. So, when you have that moment of weakness and dive face first into the cookie cake, call it what it is and move on. If you slip up for breakfast on a whim with some pancakes, don't let it determine the course of the entire day. Identify the slip-up, proactively plan the recourse to get you back in line and then stick to THAT plan. All too often, the problem lies within the moments after the slip-up, not the incident itself. Your emotions (that old monster) creep in and start informing you that "You blew it! It's all over now, absolutely no need to even consider moving forward! Man! You should just cheat for the rest of the day and call it your cheat day!" STOP! That is exactly what you are trying to correct, and it's why you are here in the first place. When the slip-up occurs (it will happen to us all, yes ALL) decide now what you will do to ensure that you implement a quick recovery. For instance, if a slip-up occurs, I may eat veggies for my lunch and eat smaller portions for my dinner. Now, I must warn you here, if this becomes habitual, you are finding more and more ways to make excuses (Rationalizing) for the slip-ups, then you my friend need to revisit the PREP FOR IT acronyms. If your Perception has been altered, it can affect how you are may Rationalize your meal decisions, which will create a false Expectation that all is well until you turn around and you find yourself back at the starting line. Every move that you make needs to be calculated and thought out. Sounds like some kind of spy novel, but anything that you proactively facilitate will pay high dividends in the long run. Just be smart. Be stealthier than your emotional monster so you can finally achieve overall weight loss and wellness that you have been desiring for years!

CHAPTER 10
Exercise: The "X" Factor

I am about to make many, many individuals extremely happy with the following statement. Exercise is not necessary for weight loss. Yeah, that's right, I said it! Now, the exercise buffs out there have a bit of steam permeating from both ears. They may have started looking for a website or social media contact to begin writing a dissertation on all of the known benefits of exercise and its association with weight loss to send to us, and I get it. Whereas my other readers, who may have a loathe-hate relationship with exercise have stepped away from the book, and can be found doing a little hallelujah hoedown in the living room, feeling like someone finally understands them! So, for the benefit of both of these groups, I will actually repeat myself here, Exercise is not necessary for weight loss (she said it again!).

However, exercise is essential to provide an environment for your overall wellness and health, and can contribute or assist in your weight loss regimen. It was great while it lasted, right?! You can establish a calorie-restricted eating plan and over time you will lose weight; however, it may come at the cost of losing some of our muscle mass in the process, which we will discuss a little later in the chapter. Exercise is the yang, to healthy eating's yin. It provides a balance to eating healthier that can contribute to a better version of yourself through the process. In this chapter, we will address a few of the misconceptions about exercise that may have been misleading. We will further discuss the benefits of incorporating exercise into your plan for overall wellness in your life and what that may look like for you specifically.

Metabolism, The Tortoise and the Hare

Our metabolism and how it functions is probably one of the touchiest, toughest topics to discuss in regards to weight loss and wellness. Metabolism is like an enigma. There are a LOT of articles, books, opinions, and myths on the subject. These have led to sheer pandemonium for individuals who want to drop a few pounds and just get a little healthier. Our metabolism is like the Wizard of Oz. It seems so vast and vague, yet, when the curtain is pulled back, it really is just a simple concept that has been over-embellished.

Let's start off by talking about your basal metabolic rate or your BMR. You may have learned about this in science class or a pre-rec class on your way to your marketing degree, but it is simply the chemical process that your body goes through to burn the energy obtained to sustain your life. Pretty straightforward, right? Now, the basal metabolic rate is simply the number of calories that a body requires to maintain normal daily functions such as heart and brain activity, and yep, I am burning just sitting here breathing! There are 3 types of metabolizing that is occurring within the body. The first is the body using energy for you to just function at a resting state, essentially just to exist. We referred to this earlier as the basal metabolic rate or BMR (60-80% of the energy consumed allocated to this). Secondly, you need energy to break down and process your food which is your energy. Say what?! Yep, that's right, you burn calories when you eat! Don't get too excited here, you really do not need all that and a bag of chips to exist, so that ship has set sail (approximately 10% of daily intake allotted to this task). The last bit of expenditure comes from your physical activity, which includes daily movements and yes, even your exercise (only 10-30% of what you consume!). Now, everyone has a different BMR, and this is where the water gets a little mucky.

Typically, your BMR is based on your height, weight, age and yes, even your gender. Some would even say that there is a familial tendency toward faster and slower metabolisms. To that I would say there is probably some validity. Growing up, I felt horrible for my sister. We are essentially the same height, same mother and father, yet we could sit down and eat a meal together, and I would struggle to gain an ounce while on the contrary, my sister would eat just a fraction of what I consumed, and she would gain before the end of the meal. It was so frustrating for her. My mother tried so many different things to attempt to increase her BMR, even attempted using over-the-counter appetite suppressants to help her with the weight loss. This truly has been such a struggle for her throughout her life. We are both females, we are essentially the same height, I was just over 2 years older than her so that was not a huge discrepancy, yet I could just breathe and lose weight. Why? What caused such a big discrepancy between the two of us? Although I was a little more physically active then she was at the time, it wasn't a factor that would be considered a game-changer. You see, that is the unknown factor for us. I was fortunate to have a faster BMR, and for many years, I was able to do very little to keep my weight down. However, without rehashing my testimony, the bill eventually comes due for us all. At some point, the age factor will catch up to us, maybe even the weight factor or a change in activity level or even the emotional factor and yes, the BMR takes a nose dive without the parachute.

So, what is my BMR Kelly, and what can I do to speed it up? Great question! If I had the exact answer to this question, you do know I would be lying on a beach somewhere just raking in the Benjamin's, right? Let's first figure out what your BMR might be before we feed your need for speed! There are many BMR calculators on-line now that will give you an idea of what your BMR is based on the data that you input from the above parameters. The BMR can change based on a number of factors, including dietary changes and even exercise. Yep, even exercise. Again, our basal metabolic rate accounts for, 60-80% of our daily energy requirements. In other words, just to breathe, have a heart rate, and think on a day-to-day basis my body will use 60-80% of its energy to provide for those functions. That is mind blowing! Unfortunately, what is even more absurd is that as a society, we have increased our caloric intake to the point that the body uses about 20-40% of what we consume for these functions, causing most of us to become overweight or even worse, obese. Obese! Kelly, are you kidding me? I can't be classified as obese, can I? The new BMI guidelines consider anyone with a BMI over 30 as obese. Sadly, this includes a large percentage of today's population. So, to this I say, if the shoe fits, well we unfortunately need to wear it (at least for now). Food is the primary fuel source and 100% (all, yes all) of the food we consume accounts for the energy that goes into our body to function. Again, remember that exercise, burns only 10-30% of these calories! Exercise accounts for a very small amount of what we expend as far as our energy consumption is concerned. I have always mentioned in teaching patients and even friends, that if we eat more than we put out in energy, we will gain weight. Could the premise be that if we eat less than we put out in energy we will lose weight? Yes, to an extent. Go back to our percentages here. We are working hard to improve 10-30% of the equation. Instead, if we focused primarily on raising the basal metabolic rate, which remember, is 60-80% of our expended energy, then the opportunity for weight loss would be far greater. I like those odds!

Let's use an example to further demonstrate this point. A woman who is approximately 5'7" in height, with a present weight of 200 pounds begins to exercise approximately 4 times a week with moderate intensity but has not implemented any caloric restrictions to the weight loss plan. Over a period of 30 days, she could experience some weight loss. If she increases her caloric intake or reduces her activities anywhere else in her life, then she stands to lose even less than that or worse, gain. That can be so disheartening to the person who puts a lot of time, energy, and funds into a gym membership or exercise class only to reap minimal dividends. However, if she implements the caloric restrictions to her eating plan along with the increase in physical activity, she is more likely to achieve her goals and feel better through the process.

Another possible issue, is when a new physical activity has been implemented, it could increase the potential of an unwanted increase in your appetite. For example, you may decide to jump on the monkey bars, or in this case, the gazelle and put some significant time and energy into that particular physical activity. This can lead to a greater desire to eat more calories or exercise a little flexibility with your food selection. Remember, when we refer back to our BMR, we are likely telling our body that it requires more fuel to produce at the new level of activity then we may actually need. Yes, when we move more, we have a tendency to eat more, whether it's because we are justifying the extra slice of pizza based on the planking, we did earlier that day, or we think that 30 minutes on the elliptical is certainly worth that piece of cake and oh yeah, I'll take seconds! Think about this for just a second. You go to the gym, get an incredible work out in, and then feeling a bit parched, you stop at the refreshment area of the gym to get a quick, cold Gatorade for the road.

STOP! Every calorie you just expended and sacrificed, can literally be cancelled out by the time you put your car in reverse and pull out of the parking spot. Yes, it even happened to me. Remember, I was doing amazing with my prepping and PREP FOR IT acronyms, seeing not only the pounds decrease but the inches as well and decided it was time to put myself back into the fitness game. Just so you know, I have a slight tendency to go to the extreme when I make a decision to do something. Exercise is no different. So, I heard about this specific HIT program that you could continue burning calories for 72 hours after working out, um where do I sign, I'm in! I started with just one time a week and built up to 2 times in a week and started feeling stronger, had more energy; but I also started getting hungrier, and I thought it would allow me to be a little more FLEXIBLE when making my eating decisions. I saw the scale and then inches go up a little and of course realized all too quickly, it happens to us all! I had to realize that just because I felt like the workouts couldn't get any more intense or difficult, it doesn't justify the need to eat more calories. Hard cookie, I mean pill, to swallow. Remember, keeping food a function is everything and has a lasting impact on your weight loss and wellness goals. I know that sounds extreme, but those little choices we make along the way can add up to big issues down the line resulting in disappointing outcomes. This part is really difficult because exercising really does increase the demand and stimulates your hunger to encourage you to increase your caloric intake. The body has never changed. It was, is, and always will be in survival mode. We are the ones who changed the rules to that game! If you choose to increase your caloric intake based on your recent change in exercise, then make sure that the right choices in foods and calories have been considered to avoid this, all too common pitfall with exercise.

Again, if I was a betting individual, I would play the odds. So, it seems that the likely role that exercise plays with weight loss is to create an environment that will accelerate our metabolism so that we can use the 60-80% to our advantage. Industries have made millions off of you and I over this very topic. There are supplements, patches, teas and even coffees that tout an ability to increase your metabolism without any obvious effort on your part. If it smells like a fish, jumps like a fish and flops like one, remember… it's a fish. If it sounds too good to be true….it probably is. We need to use exercise as an accelerator to speed up the basal metabolic rate, so that we can do what we do best, and that is just function. Avoid getting caught up into gimmicks and schemes that offer amazing solutions and a marked increase in your metabolism simply by taking the little blue pill once a day. Really? That's all it will take? Well, if that were so, we would all be living the skinny life then wouldn't we?

The National Center for Health Statistics estimates that between 2015 and 2016, the obesity rate (BMI over 30) was 39.8 percent of adults over the age of 20, and 7 ½ percent of those were markedly obese. An additional 30% were considered overweight. This doesn't seem like rocket science to me, but based on these percentages over 70% of our country is presently suffering from eating more than we are putting out in energy. That is staggering! The worst part about all of this is that the numbers are predicted to continue rising within the next decade. Enter you. You may not be able to change that percentage as a whole, but you can change one number in that figure and that is your contribution to the percentage. You can make the difference that is needed for you.

So, what are some methods to enhance or accelerate our present BMR rate? A higher BMR has several advantages. It allows us to burn calories easier and, in turn, can assist, and I use this term loosely, in achieving our weight loss goals. It can also give us an energy boost and provide an overall feeling of wellness. In doing so, it can give us additional enthusiasm for prepping and following our eating plan, which gives us the momentum to want to exercise more. Then when we start to see those amazing results, you guessed it?! You have now created your own positive feedback system that can continue to work in your favor, albeit as long as you continue to move in the right direction! Exercise and eating well contribute to improved sleep patterns and an overall sense of well-being, again feeding into the system we would like to see working for us on a daily basis.

One of the biggest ways to boost the BMR is to increase your intake of proteins. Hello?! There is a thermic effect that we get from eating food. In other words, it takes more calories to burn and digest some foods than others. Protein sources like beef, poultry, fish, eggs, and some dairy products will increase the metabolic rate for digestion by 15-30%, compared to only 5-10% for carbohydrates and less than 1% for fats. If you have ever eaten a steak or a burger and feel that you haven't even started to digest after several hours of eating the meal, you are experiencing the need for a greater thermal effect to burn this particular energy source. I think of this a lot like the gas that you may put in your car, the regular unleaded is cheaper (so are most carbs on the shelf) but not as healthy for the car as the premium unleaded (burns more efficiently). For my patients that suffer with metabolic conditions such as Insulin Resistance (IR) or Polycystic Ovarian Syndrome (PCOS), I strongly urge them to follow a link and balance plan. In this plan, you should balance the protein to carbohydrates at a ratio of 15 grams of protein to 30 grams of carbohydrates, with no more than 30 grams of carbs at a sitting.

I have simplified this by simply instructing them to remember a 2:1 ratio of carbohydrate to protein, making food choices easier. In fact, I further instruct them that they can have a protein without a carbohydrate because for them, their metabolism is far worse than for the average person. They don't even get the chance to burn the food source as an energy if the carbohydrate intake is substantial. They will simply store it as a fat, and the body will just move on from there. An additional advantage to eating more proteins is it will typically cause you to stay fuller longer, allowing you to eat fewer calories in the course of the day. This can even contribute to less muscle loss with a calorie restricted eating plan.

Increasing your intake of water has also been shown to cause a short-term rise in our BMR. Studies have noted that drinking at least 16 ounces of water every 3-4 hours can increase your overall BMR by 10-30% when done consistently throughout the day. So, Kelly what you're telling me is, I can raise my metabolic rate simply by drinking water? It may not be a game-changer, but remember, small changes over a long period of time create amazing results. So, you may hit the restrooms a little more often than before, but at least you are doing a little preventive medicine by keeping the bladder flushed and healthy as well! Drinking water before sitting down to eat a meal can also give you the sensation of feeling fuller and reducing caloric intake even further. Again, every little bit makes a difference in the long run.

Yes, high intensity (HIT) workouts have been shown to raise the metabolic rate not just during the workout, but for many of these programs, they continue to force the body to metabolize at a higher rate, for sometimes hours after the workout is over. Additionally, HIT workouts allow you to burn more fat, thus reducing the fat composition of the body over time. WOW! That means that there is essentially a win/win that is occurring just by engaging in HIT workouts. Another advantage of high intensity work outs, is increasing muscle mass throughout the body that will require more energy to just function. You guessed it! It will increase your BMR to accommodate the new demand from the body, as muscle requires more from the body to routinely function than any other parts or systems in the body. This is notable, as well, with weight lifting programs that allow you to retain muscle mass while attempting weight loss simultaneously. When this occurs, less muscle mass is lost thus allowing our bodies to continue to function at a higher BMR. Many individuals who embark on a weight loss journey without doing any weight lifting or training may find a decrease in overall muscle mass and a slight reduction to their BMR. Yep, there are advantages to implementing exercise into your overall wellness goals.

Another factor that potentially improves or enhances your BMR is sleep. This is what many individuals call their "sweet spot." Sleeping helps my metabolism, Kelly? "Well, then sign me up because this happened to be my major in college. I was going pro until I had to get a job!" All joking aside, loss of sleep has had a negative impact on the function of our metabolism, and has also been shown to increase the risk for insulin resistance and even increased blood sugar levels in the body that can lead to Type II Diabetes. Obviously, this doesn't happen overnight, excuse the pun, but if you don't allow for adequate rest, over time the body will start to respond negatively. It has even been shown to increase the hunger hormone, ghrelin (think growling or hunger) and decrease the fullness hormone leptin, hence increasing the probability for weight gain. This can begin to contribute to the positive feedback loop in a negative way, and we don't have time for all of that!

Increasing the medium chain fats in your diet can also contribute to a rise in your overall BMR. One fat that has the highest composite of medium chain fats is coconut oil and can easily be substituted in many recipes to offer healthier, higher functioning options. Because of its unique makeup, coconut oil has been shown to be beneficial in assisting in weight loss. No, I am not saying if you switch to using only coconut oil you will lose weight. What I am suggesting is making small changes, over a long period of time can contribute to amazing success. Sound familiar?

Another contributing factor is doing away with the 3 larger meals and substituting 5-6 smaller meals to allow the body to operate in a more continuous thermal effect especially if these foods are protein or of a higher protein content. Just remember, anytime we eat, it causes the body to go into work-mode to break the food down into energy; however, it does not mean we get to eat king cake (it's the season) or cupcakes because we are in a constant energy-burning state. This is probably one of the down sides to the intermittent fasting that has been a recent hit for those dieting professionals. When we do not eat, the body initially burns but then can inadvertently slow based on the lack of demand. Another potential pitfall with this eating plan is when an individual comes off of the recent fasting episode without solid discipline, they will eat whatever and as much as they want of a food that may not be the best option for weight loss. So, discipline is essential with that particular eating plan, for that matter any eating plan.

Eating more whole foods has a definite advantage to increasing your overall BMR. Why is this? It takes a lot more for our bodies to process a whole carrot than a pureed carrot in a soup. A sweet potato has far more fiber than a sweet potato chip. Steel cut oats have more fiber and more thermal demand than the oatmeal that you will find in the cardboard boxes. They have literally been stripped down to make it easier to cook but also easier to digest. Therefore, you guessed it, they require less thermal energy to break the food down. The old adage that says "we are what we eat" truly hits the nail on the head. Organic, unprocessed foods that are whole grained or in a raw form are going to be far more difficult for the body to process than a cupcake or chocolate shake. When I teach the PCOS class at our facility, I talk about how we have changed as "consumers." We used to eat far more whole foods: foods made from scratch that had tons of fiber packed in them.

Fast forward to our present day, and we have essentially become what I like to call "cardboard eaters." A significant amount of the food consumed in our society is packaged in either a cardboard box or bag and takes very little effort to prepare for consumption. This can only mean one thing. The food manufacturer boasts that the meal is even easier than before to prepare. With that being said, it can result in our bodies more readily absorbing that same meal. As a result, it will take less effort for the body to burn the food as an energy source. Subsequently, the body is forced to store the fuel as a fat to use at a later date. Swell, huh?!

Another extremely important factor that directly affects our resting BMR is reducing the stress we have in our life. We will cover this in more detail in the next chapter, but when we stress, our bodies opt to trigger a survival mechanism in the body that will, you guessed it, slow down our metabolism to protect the body. You have heard the saying, don't sweat the small stuff? Well, when you reduce your stress, you are not only positively affecting your BMR, but stress is one of the major triggers in our PREP FOR IT acronyms that will cause us to emotionally eat in the first place. Fix what you have the ability to fix, but if it is out of your control, then fretting over it will not change the outcome.

So Kelly, what about exercise? Tips, pointers, anything? Our ultimate goal is to develop a plan for overall wellness and weight loss. We spent many chapters equipping you with tools and resources to help you reach those weight loss goals, but weight loss does not always equate to wellness. That's where exercise comes in. Exercise can provide a platform for our bodies to start performing more proficiently and healthier than they have. Not only does this make our metabolism run at a higher rate, but also provide the needed environment to improve sleep, reduce stress, and even postpone or reverse chronic disease conditions. Think of exercise as the best medicine you can take. It will cost you just a little sweat, and maybe a few tears, but can certainly make you feel better when you have finished.

What can I do to incorporate exercise into my wellness program, and how much would be considered enough? Absolutely great questions. There are a few not so scientific suggestions that I have for you in regard to exercise and implementing this into your wellness plan. Just do it! Take the first step, jump, or plank. None of this is as relevant as just doing something. Anything that increases your heart rate for at least 20-30 minutes, 3-4 times in a week will have a positive impact over time when consistently incorporated into your routine. For Pete's sake, just do something fun! The worst thing in the world you could do is start an exercise program that you loathe. If it bores you to tears, then move on to something else. Enjoy the time that you are working out or getting fit; this will create the positive momentum that you are striving to achieve. Not to mention, when you find something you enjoy, it will make it easier to commit to the goal of getting it done! Classes that you can participate in with other like-minded individuals can become a motivator to pursue additional physical activities and goals that can further your wellness and weight loss goals. If you like ka-ra-te, then by all means join a dojo and let the good times roll! You have an affinity to boxing and beating up something? Then get a bag or join a boxing gym; you never know, you may unearth a hidden talent to rock and roll with the speed bag. Your preference may be more in line with power yoga. Then, by all means, get into that dolphin pose and get to work! I am not particularly fond of indoor cycling. I know for many, this has become an obsession, but for me…ehhh. But with the recent pandemic, we were forced to put together a makeshift gym in our home. With limited space for the equipment, we opted for a recumbent bike. Now, I know what most of you are thinking. "Look, she went and bought herself an indoor clothes line, because for many, their bikes become a convenient means to hang-dry a few clothes. In order to make this exercise enticing, I searched online for 30-minute videos that provided scenic paths to ride my virtual bike. There are hundreds of free options and you get to take "a ride" in all parts of the world! Now I find myself looking through the videos to find a really cool location and hurry home to hop on the bike and peddle through the streets of rural Italy! Failing to find the fun in exercise can cause us to get disenfranchised far too quickly. So, change your routines up, consider even changing the location of the workout. Since writing this book, I have been blessed to incorporate a commercial-grade treadmill into our home gym. I am able to follow along with the trainer while hiking, walking or running through different parts of the world. Now, that has been a game-changer! Many of these things will play a major role in your long-term success with your wellness and weight loss journey.

I know that I have provided a strong viewpoint as to why exercise is only marginally responsible for weight loss, but remember, if you put out more energy than you consume in calories, it will certainly contribute to an eventual weight loss. Again remember, we paint the barn door until the paint sticks. Persistent consistency will eventually provide tangible results. The common thread through all of this is just do something to get moving, and keep moving, and those small incidental changes will lead to big differences that will create amazing results.

CHAPTER 11

"The Game-changer" Emotional Health and Well-being

A famous character once said, "Worrying won't stop the bad stuff from happening; it just stops you from enjoying the good." He also noted that, "In the book of life, the answers aren't in the back." Another one that absolutely stole my heart was, "All you really need is love, but a little chocolate now and then doesn't hurt." He was a lovable loser who was created to represent the traits and even flaws in the average person. If you haven't quite guessed yet, I am referring to the iconic character, Charlie Brown. When we allow the bad stuff to take precedence in our lives, then we have very little left to focus on what is truly good. In the comic strip developed and illustrated by Charles M. Schulz, the main character Charlie, was an innocent and meek child who experienced a bit of suffering in his life and showed the readers how he handled the daunting, daily obstacles that he typically encountered. Even though bullied and made out to be a "loser," he was a gutsy and determined kid who overcame many difficulties along the way. Was he perfect? Not on your life! He exhibited so many traits that you see in each and every one of us: the good, the bad, and yes, even the ugly. His posse, was no exception. Lucy, Linus, Peppermint Pattie, and his loyal companion, Snoopy covered the gamut of emotions, personalities, and flaws that we all exhibit. Still, in each and every one of us lies the ability to see the best in others and the best in ourselves. One thing we must strive to do in this PREP FOR IT process is to find a place where we are happy with our progress, the results, and the person that we have become in the process.

At this point in our journey, you have probably already started to work on a prep strategy and a schedule that will work for you, as well as walking through the PREP FOR IT process. You may have even identified your specific triggers and what your expectations should be in this process. You have even purchased your supplies and gone through extreme efforts to ensure that you stay focused on the long-term plan and what that entails. What brings all of this together in a nice package for you to carry through the course of your life is to understand how your emotional health plays a major role in the entire process. I know, we talked about the emotional monster and how his ultimate goal is to wreak havoc on our lives as much and as often as he can. I know we have worked through the PREP FOR IT process to equip you with the tools that can help you to generate positive momentum and success in your wellness and weight loss goals. However, without thoroughly understanding the true role of emotional health, I am giving you this large, beautiful house, wonderfully landscaped without a key to get in. So, we will spend the next chapter talking about the importance of balance in our lives, the art of saying "NO," realizing that we are awesome with all of our imperfections, and providing the key to finally move forward.

Mental Health and the effects of having a mental health illness are not foreign concepts to the United States. According to the National Alliance on Mental Illness, 47.6 million people suffer from some form of mental illness. This equates to about 1 in every 5 adults in 2018. That number is staggering to me. Even more astounding, these statistics fail to reflect the number of individuals who chose to avoid seeking treatment. They may hide behind their illness, or in our case donuts, maybe even attempting to overcompensate for what they are feeling. Public service announcements noting that "You are NOT alone," have been published, simply because the number of people directly or indirectly affected by this, is noteworthy. Furthermore, one study found that 50% of women and 41% who suffered from a serious mental illness, also were dealing with obesity and being overweight according to the Obesity Action Coalition. Did the obesity cause the mental disrepair, or did the mental disorders and undue stress cause the obesity? This is a true case of which came first, the chicken or the egg? Going all the way back to how WE got here in the first place, we know that this is a feedback system that, if allowed, will run amuck in our lives. So, does mental health play a role in your long-term success with wellness and weight loss? Absolutely! We just spent several chapters solidifying this point. We want to further implement strategies that close down for good, the steep slope of emotional eating that we have traveled on in the past. We are starting a new journey, where we are just as good to our self as we are to everyone else! In all honesty, this takes as much effort and planning as it does to prep for the week.

We want you to get to a point in this journey where you are not having to revisit the PREP FOR IT acronyms on a weekly basis. Rather, they become standard guidelines for you to apply intermittently as needed through the course of your life. Every time I see the word guidelines, it makes me think of the movie, "Pirates of the Caribbean." The captain said they are not pirate rules but more like "guidelines" (stated in my best pirate accent!). When our ship gets off course, we can simply walk back through those steps to get ship-shape and back to smooth sailing again.

A Psychology Today article written by The Squeaky Wheel author, Guy Winch, PhD., discusses the 7 habits of highly emotionally healthy individuals, how to identify triggers in our life and put some proactive measures in place. We spend a significant amount of time working on our physical health, but often neglect our emotional fitness and the obvious needs we have to improve its current state. The basis of the steps, are to find the self-defeating behaviors that lie within us, and in laymen terms, put a beat-down on them. We want to finally create resolutions to minimize the control these behaviors have in our lives. Now, this is easier said than done, but when you realize that your emotional health is directly tied to how you treat and care for yourself physically, then the prepping and preparing will also become just a function, a mechanism to produce the best version of ourselves.

First things first

We must be able to identify negative triggers in our lives, not only to avoid dealing with the emotional monster, but also to allow us to obtain the best version of ourselves. Negative triggers can lead to the most toxic, brutal state that too many people call "home sweet home." This is stress. Stress is probably the most significant issue that our world deals with today. It has become a powerful catalyst to anxiety, depression, obesity, and other mental health disorders. Even worse, it can lead to suicide. When we are exposed to acute stress, our body releases hormones that create physical changes like increasing our blood pressure, making the brain more alert, our muscles more tense, and even increasing our pulse. Now I am not implying that all stress is bad. In fact, short bursts of stress can be positive, like when you are walking in the woods and you realize that you are being followed by a large furry animal with big claws who may have just found his way out of hibernation. That kind of stress works in your favor! I want my muscles to stand in attention, my pulse to tell me something is wrong, and my brain to tell me to get out of there and I mean quick! That kind of stress is therapeutic and helpful to the situation we are facing. Ongoing chronic stress however, causes prolonged frustration, anger, or nervousness. When not sufficiently handled, it can lead to both physical and mental illness. Think about it. The same physical changes occur, but now the blood pressure stays high longer. The rapid pulse persists, and the muscles stay tense far too long, creating an environment that can lead to chronic changes such as high blood pressure, diabetes, heart disease, and you guessed it, obesity.

Now I have to say I hate this analogy! I really do, but it is truly the best way to explain how stress, grief, or any negative emotion can affect us both physically and mentally. When lightning strikes an object or individual, it has an entry and must have an exit. It is an electrical current that travels. Essentially it will meander through the object until it can find a successful exit, likely damaging anything in its path. In this case, stress or any other negative emotion for that matter, is very similar. When you deal with a stressful event or lifestyle without an outlet of some sort, then that negative emotion will wreak havoc throughout the body, taking on many different forms. Many people suffer from stomach disorders such as ulcers, reflux, or irritable bowel syndrome because they internalize their stressors. I tell people I don't care what they do to process their stressors and negative feelings; it can be cross-stitching, kick-boxing, or whatever as long as they find something to allow the negative emotions to be released out of the body. I have a tendency to vacillate toward something I am able to beat-up on to help redirect the stress (boxing bag, volleyball, tennis ball, etc.). Finding something that allows you to compartmentalize what is agonizing to you will provide the much-needed relief that keeps your stress levels low and your positive attitude strong and resilient.

Getting to the point where we are not allowing the small occurrences during the course of the day to affect us, will pay huge dividends in preventing stress. Prolonged stress has the potential to lead to anxiety. In translation, don't sweat the small stuff! My husband and I often talk about the movies that we allow to run in our minds. In fact, reruns will occur over and over again if we allow them. If we don't curtail them, the movies can lead to cliffhangers and plot twists that have absolutely no chance of happening. All because we allow our minds to take charge and jump off the deep end. When I am confronted with a stressful situation, I think, what is the worst thing that can happen? If it is not life-altering or physically damaging, I simply tell myself to get over it and stop worrying about it. I know this is easier said than done. This is something that takes training and repetition, much like prepping and proactively planning helps deter us from binging on cupcakes simply because we have an extreme issue or emotion that we are facing. Using our PREP FOR IT steps can go a long way in not only minimizing our reactive food choices, but also helping us to take control of the stressors which can create further obstacles in our weight loss and wellness journey.

One of the best ways to reduce the stressors in your life is to figure out the trigger and work on removing it from your life. Again, this is easier said than done, but often we insist on staying in a situation that provides a major source of negative energy simply because we think it may take too much effort to do a deep cleaning in the corners of our own world. A bad job that you simply loathe? Look, a job is a job. If it were pure joy, then we would say we are going to joy today, right? The job that you choose to accept and therefore perform should provide some feeling of accomplishment, gratification, and a level of success no matter what your work looks like. If your job is creating such significant stress that you binge eat your way through the kitchen at night to cope, then by all means start looking for a new one! Life is too short to stay stagnant simply because change seems daunting. By no means is this a recommendation to walk into your boss's office, throw down the deuces, and peace out on a Monday morning, but if this is a significant source of stress contributing to reactive choices and a downward spiral with no end in sight, then start-up the think tank. What would you LOVE to do, how could you get there, and what type of planning and resources would it take to make the change?

Toxic People Syndrome

Having toxic people as part of your life can create unnecessary stress. Do I think they can benefit from help and someone willing to listen and care about their needs? Sure! However, not at the expense of YOUR health or wellness. Negative doom and gloom individuals will suck the wind out of your sails faster than a freight train going down a steep hill. Recognize them, put a plan in place to ensure they don't monopolize your time, and start introducing more positive influences into your life. Now, if YOU happen to suffer from what I like to call the Eeyore syndrome, then consider doing introspection on what is causing you to feel and act this way. Eliciting some changes could get you on the road to a better version of you! In the article discussing 7 habits of highly emotionally healthy people, Dr. Winch mentions a disruption of the urge to brood, or relive all the occurrences that caused you to feel the way that you do. By disrupting the cycle of reliving the tale day in and day out, you are creating a new habit of dealing with the issues, moving on, and creating opportunities for more positive influences in your life. He mentions things like choosing activities that can distract us, allow us to compartmentalize and close the chapter on the event, thereby avoiding an environment of constant worry or pessimism.

There are many individuals who have what we call co-dependency. They actually feel better when there is someone who needs and relies on them to continuously function and will often complain about the situation that we, in fact, have created. Overall, this is not a healthy relationship because without good balance and an ability to identify when enough is enough, you, my friend, are on slippery slope back to visit your old friend, the emotional monster and his buffet of binge eating. If there is some part of you that can identify with this particular behavior, create opportunities to be able to step away and re-group, allowing you to avoid the potential for emotional turmoil to become the mainstay.

The Balancing Act

A very long time ago, I had a brief stent in the Education Department of a hospital in Louisiana and developed and taught a program on "The Balancing Act." I remember putting the program together and teaching it to fellow employees in the hospital and realizing, I wasn't really practicing what I was preaching. I mean teaching! Fast forward, and I now find myself teaching on the very same topic, almost every single day. However, with experience comes wisdom. By realizing you need to turn off the stressors (job, school, extra-curricular activities, etc.) This can be challenging to achieve, but when you get just a tiny taste of how effective balance can be in your life, then you are motivated to find permanent ways to achieve it. One of my main mantras to ask patients is simply, "Do you want to give the best of you, or the rest of you?" The response to my questions, include: a look of stupor as they are mulling over this question and an appropriate response, a well of tears developing in their eyes as the realization of that question hits home, or a dissertation on all of the reasons they do NOT have time to do anything for themselves because life is just too busy! Look, I totally get it! Life is busy for all of us, and our society today would like to make you feel like a lightweight if you are unable to do 14 things at one time, and oh yes, please make sure everything is perfect as well! The illustration I use to make the point even further, is utilizing the flight attendants' instructions to you before you take off and hit 30,000 feet. "In the event we experience an altitude change, your oxygen may drop from the ceiling, please put the mask on you first and then assist anyone around you with their masks." Why? Because without the necessary oxygen required to breathe, you my friend, are essentially one large human paperweight, worthless to anyone around you.

So, I ask the question…Do you want to give the best of you or the rest of you? New mothers and moms who have their hands full with a couple of little ones can relate all too well to this question. They always want to give the best of themselves, but guilt all too often finds its way into their hearts long enough to squash any thoughts of doing something that provides some stress relief let alone pleasure. When you are able to get the epiphany that spending about 30 minutes a few times a week on something by yourself that you thoroughly enjoy, can allow you to give everyone around you the best version of yourself, you would jump in feet first!

Think about our lives like we are carrying 2 large water pails full of issues, those that are dumped onto us and the things that are taken from us (I like the visual of the woman who carries the two pails of water on a large pole over her back). One of those pails, if not emptied by a hobby or activity that can release the stressors, will overflow. We will lash out to others around us. The other bucket gives everything we've got to those closest to us. If not replenished, we will have nothing to give which creates further imbalance. You need the hobbies that have only your name on them just as much as the Calgon moments and date night with no strings attached. Both provide you with an avenue to create balance in your life, which in turn minimizes the need to find comfort in the ice cream section of your local supermarket.

Eye of the Tiger

Getting rid of the "all or nothing mentality" is absolutely critical to your ability to achieve long-term success with your wellness and weight loss goals. All too often, when we do not reach the initial goal that we have set for ourselves, we become very critical, and if not careful, have the potential to completely derail our train of success. Progress is still forward movement toward the ultimate goal, no matter how small or large it may seem. We need to become our biggest fan. It's not necessary to get arrogant and full of ourselves, but we need to be able to readily celebrate the small victories in the journey so this marathon of wellness and weight loss can become the success we originally envisioned. Don't compare yourself to the person next to you! The biggest threat to your success is looking to the right or the left when you take this journey. In horse racing, if they are concerned about the focus of a particular horse, the trainers will put blinders on the outside of their eyes so they literally see only the dirt track in front of them, unable to focus on who is running to the right or the left of them. If you are faced with distractions from those around you, it may be necessary to slap the blinders on and focus on just your progress, allowing you to reach the success you desire. Sometimes, the worst thing in the world is when a couple will start a weight loss and wellness journey together. Now if you have any notion of how this works, you wouldn't ever agree to participate in it. When a husband and wife attempt the same eating plan or physical training together, it is inevitable that the male will lose weight faster, tone up quicker with little to no effort, and this can be very disheartening to his counterpart. Stick to your lane, your goals, and your progress! YOU are your toughest competition, so when you see progress, take time to celebrate the small wins that give you momentum to conquer the bigger goals that you have set.

Say What?

Taking the journey for overall wellness and weight loss can be stressful, painful, and sometimes even lonely. Many around you will continue to go on with life with not a care in the world, celebrating each and every small accomplishment with a tasty treat, all while you are doing everything within your power to just achieve some positive momentum. It's great to take the time to celebrate the small wins and create the positive momentum, but having an unbiased individual, who you can trust to be candid with you may be your most powerful weapon in the war for wellness and weight loss.

Going back to my testimony chapter, I talked about how I became an emotional eater, and what led me to rely on food to comfort me through a tumultuous situation. I mentioned that I would eat whoppers and hot tamale candy even if the television wasn't on while my husband quietly watched this horror movie unfold with little control over the outcome. Yes, he could have spoken up and simply said, "Are you really going to eat that big box of whoppers for dinner?" but at the time, that episode may not have ended happily ever after. That had to be difficult to witness. Like a car wreck that you can see happening from the passenger's seat. Yet pressing the floorboard on your side has no effect on the outcome. In a situation such as this, you need an accountability partner who can discuss the tough topics with you and give you a little glass check when they think you need it without the fear of the wrath that you may unleash. You have to be open to constructive feedback and realize that your accountability partner is there to help you succeed and assist you in making the tough choices to achieve the overall goal. This can be a mentor, spouse, a counterpart who you work with and trust, or even a loyal friend. No matter who you feel is best suited to become your Robin in this Batman journey, make sure you give them safe ground to land and say the hard things you may need to hear. When you need them the most, allow them the opportunities to speak up without fear of getting verbally pummeled in the process!

When I think of creating an atmosphere that promotes optimum mental health, I realize that life happens, and no matter how much planning takes place, the inevitable will occur. You may lose a job, require a major surgery, or yes, lose a loved one suddenly. You may find yourself feeling all of those familiar emotions that brought you here in the first place. We talked about this before. Plan for the disasters so that you have a plan in place when they occur. This is far easier to say than to actually implement. Kelly, how do I plan for the death of a loved one? I truly wish I had the answer for you. Unfortunately, I don't have the answer, and it has happened to me more than I would care to say. However, knowing that I have identified what brought me to the place of emotional eating and led me to become overweight somehow makes it a bit easier to address. Making sure to have healthy measures in place to cope with the downfalls that will inevitably occur to us all, goes a long way in the success we will ultimately achieve. I will provide more commentary on this topic in the afterthoughts of the book.

The Lost Art of "NO!"

I literally could write an entire chapter on how saying NO more can contribute to a better mental outlook. We have become a "yes" society. This not only pressures us into doing more things in less time, but we also live in fear of disappointing those who ask the questions in the first place. We get asked to work on school, work, and community projects, and if we dare answer with that little 2-letter dirty word, we are made to feel inept and labeled a slacker. Saying NO more often to some things that may not be game changers for you, can be the biggest liberating measure you put in place during this entire process. We are gifted with 24 hours each and every day, the Lord willing. Using more discretion when determining where that time will be allocated will provide more balance and allow you to devote more effort to the things that matter most in your life. It allows you to give the best of you, not the rest of you!

S.O.S

What about the anxiety and depression I already have? How do I adequately address this so that it doesn't become a barrier to my success? Many individuals who find themselves overweight may have gotten there because of a situational stressor in their lives. The problem is, once we develop anxiety and depression, it has to be addressed and managed to provide a platform for true success to be achieved. Speaking with a counselor or psychologist can be extremely beneficial in providing a therapeutic environment for healing and recovery and should not be frowned upon or create a negative stigma for you in any way. If I had the flu or I was having severe back pain, other than whining about it to my spouse, I would make an appointment to see the medical provider to get an idea of what am I dealing with so that I can recover and get back to optimum health.

Why is this such a difficult concept to understand when we are faced with an emotional disorder that may have developed over time or as a result of a trying experience in our life? Think of the title of this section, S.O.S. It is imperative for your overall success to find a place that is safe (S) to discuss the sensitive issues. An open (O) environment void of judgement or criticism, and that can provide a level of security (S) to share your personal concerns and issues. Seeking help with an emotional disorder is the strongest decision you could make and the smartest solution to ultimately achieving long term success. There are licensed counselors who specialize in many different mental and emotional disorders, including many eating disorders. Finding the one that is right for you is essential in creating an optimum atmosphere for emotional wellness.

Our emotional health plays a major role in our overall success in this journey, so before strapping up for the long haul, do an inventory of what your mental health looks like and what may need revision to create a greater environment for success. Strength isn't determined by what we have, or for that matter, what may be lacking, but, on the contrary, it is found in our weaknesses that are identified and addressed. Here is where we tap into our greatest potential and strength that we didn't think we truly had. As you review the steps in the PREP FOR IT process, start formulating a plan of action for your wellness and weight loss goals. Please take the time to reflect on any emotional barriers you possess that could be obstacles to reaching your final destination in this journey. I'm not sure we really ever get to the final destination. There are things we will constantly review and evaluate, tweak here and there to improve the process. Just remember to bloom where you are planted. Get the most out of your plan and your life, and create the positive feedback system in your own life!

PART III

From Soup to Nuts: PREP FOR IT
6-Week Starter Course

Assembly Required

Man's greatest successes were not accomplished simply by getting up one morning and deciding to climb to the peak of Mount Everest, or develop an innovative new mode of travel like flying. No, our greatest triumphs as a collective body were achieved when there was a simple idea, followed by a plethora of conceptual plans that led to a strategically developed process to reach the established goal. That is where the Resource Chapter of PREP FOR IT came into fruition. It's one thing to give you an outline of what can assist you in meeting your wellness and weight loss goals. However, it is a whole other ball of wax to provide some step-by-step guidelines that can provide the best opportunity for success. Am I stating that the resource chapter has all the soup-to-nuts YOU may need to reach your established goals? Absolutely not! What I am telling you is that with a simple idea (I want to lose 25 pounds), a plethora of conceptual plans (PREP FOR IT acronyms and the resource chapter), you can strategically develop the process whereby you obtain the established goal.

In many of the chapters of the book, we provided hands-on exercises, to be completed at the time, allowing you, to essentially eat the frog. What?! Did she really say that? Yes, yes, I did! *Eat That Frog* is a book written by Brian Tracy reviewing 21 ways to stop procrastinating and get more done in less time. Whenever I am trying to accomplish a large task or prepare for a big event, I develop a plan, but when I review the steps in the plan, I am looking at the areas that will be potential road-blocks for me. Things that make doing the dishes seem like a night on the town! When I identify my road-blocks, I muster up the courage and get them done first. In Brian Tracy's book, he explains that "Mark Twain once said if the first thing you do each morning is eat a live frog, then you could go through the rest of the day with the satisfaction of knowing that it is probably the worst thing you will do throughout the day!" By providing activities in the supplemental workbook specific to each chapter, we essentially wanted to set the table, and serve YOUR frog on our finest China. In essence, help you eat your own frog.

However, to really ensure that we provided the resources to you for the greatest success, we put together a more comprehensive plan of sorts that will give you detailed activities to assist with your plan of attack. Something that you could continue to refer back to from time to time when needed. Whatever the case may be, we wanted to have an ongoing resource that was quick, easy to work through, and provided all the tools you would need to start your journey for wellness and weight loss.

You, are finally here. After working through the PREP FOR IT acronyms, you have figured out what the emotional monster is doing in your life, and you have started to implement strategies to boot him to the curve. There are many great eating plans on the market. Ultimately, finding the plan that best suits your lifestyle, current schedule, and financial means, will provide a successful foundation to reach your wellness and weight loss goals. I want to help. It can be daunting at times, to figure out the best way to achieve your desired results, and having a little help along the way can be a game changer.

The purpose of the 6-week Start-Up course is to provide a turn-key plan enabling you to embark on your weight loss and wellness journey without having to reinvent the wheel, sail, and motor for your trip. No, I will not have groceries delivered to your door (although you can certainly make arrangements to do that!). I wanted to provide a foundation for you to develop your proactive planning and re-establish some good habits along the way. Will you have to work? Ah, yes! Anything worth obtaining will come at the cost of some sweat equity. However, in order to facilitate this process, I have set up a 6-week course that includes 5 main meals and 5 sides (2 servings each) to be eaten through the course of the week for lunch and dinner. I have included a grocery list, detailed recipes and a guideline for each prep week, to help you navigate this process. Essentially, we wanted to take any decision-making issues out of the equation, thereby allowing you to acclimate to the proactive process.

The PREP FOR IT 6-week start-up course is set up to be utilized with the book, however the course can be completed independently from the book. Remember, if you are a novice in the kitchen, the Essentials 101 video (www.prep4it.com) allows you to learn tools of the trade that will make this process far easier, and contribute to your overall success. If an instruction manual offers the reader the opportunity to successfully assemble a piece of furniture, how much more will the starter course benefit you with your wellness and weight loss goals. Think of this like one, big instruction manual helping to build a brand new healthier, happier you.

Start-Up Guidelines (Remember to say this in your best pirate voice!)

- Make sure to take a few hours prior to the next week and plan out your prep process.
- Drink at least 6-8 large glasses (6-8 ounces) of water a day (if needed get the water bottle that coaches you through this.)
- First week of the PREP FOR IT Start-Up Course, remove all soft drinks and sweet beverages from your eating plan (this includes any artificial sweeteners that can falsely elevate your insulin levels in the body).
- Allow yourself 1 healthy snack a day. (Refer to our snack list on our essentials page.)
- You can have an unlimited amount of salad and veggies for the next 6 weeks. (Refrain from using any high-calorie dressings or sauces. I want your calories to count!)
- Schedule your time to food prep each week either in your phone or calendar and stick with the schedule. (This can often be the most difficult guideline to follow.)
- At the end of each week, work through the PEER process. (Prep, Eat, Evaluate, Repeat).

- Let this become engrained in your weekly routines. I promise you will thank me for this one later!)
- Avoid the temptation to work outside of the lines (try to stick with the recipes and suggested foods as much as possible to allow for your greatest success).
- During the first 6 weeks of the plan, use the smart phone apps to help you count daily calories to ensure you are not exceeding between 1100-1200 Calories/day.
- Focus on a weight loss goal of 1/2 - 1 pound per week. With this goal, you are looking at 3-6 pounds in 6 weeks, and if you can maintain this momentum, in 1 year you will have lost between 26 and 52 pounds. (Game-changer!)
- Have fun! (We all have a choice on how we see things; if we see an adventure, well, that is exactly what we will get! However, if we look at this as another chore, you will get that as well.)

6 Week Start-Up Course Overview

Week One

- Carne Verde with Roasted Mashed Cauliflower
- Sausage and Peppers with Caramelized Butternut Squash
- Roasted Chicken Wings, Baked Sweet Potato, and Roasted Broccoli
- Tequila Sunrise Salmon with Parmesan/Garlic Zoodles and Asparagus
- Eggroll in a Bowl with Homemade Kale Chips

Week Two

- Beef and Broccoli with Cauliflower Rice
- Honey Mustard Baked Chicken, Hasselbeck new Potatoes and Ratatouille
- Korean Beef Lettuce Wraps with Asian Brussel Sprout Slaw
- Buffalo Chicken Salad with Homemade Ranch Dressing over Mixed Greens and Ratatouille
- Pecan Crusted Trout/Catfish with Mushroom Pilaf Cauliflower Rice and Sautéed Green Beans

Week Three

- Everything Bagel Pan-Fried Trout/Cod with Baked Sweet Potato
- Chicken Enchiladas with Turmeric/Lime/Cilantro Rice
- Bacon Mushroom Burger and Zucchini Parmesan Fries
- Smothered Pork chops with Mushrooms and Onions and Sweet Potato Mash
- Combination Fried Rice with Sautéed Asian Cabbage

Week Four

- Chicken Shawarma, Turmeric/Pine Nut Cauliflower Rice and Cucumber Salad
- Best Meatloaf Ever, Roasted Yellow Beets and Roasted Mashed Cauliflower
- Sausage and Chicken Jambalaya, Broccoli
- Miso Tuna Bowl
- Pork BBQ Ribs/Sweet Potato Fries and Roasted Okra or Green Beans

Week Five

- Bolognese Meat Sauce with Roasted Spaghetti Squash or Palm Noodles
- Pistachio and Pork Rind Panko Crusted Salmon with Avocado Salad
- Barbacoa Beef with Fixins and Sweet Potato Mash
- Mongolian Chicken with Cauliflower Rice and Green Beans
- Swedish Meatballs with Roasted Butternut Squash

Week Six

- Stuffed Peppers with Roasted Brussel Sprouts and Bacon
- Chicken Cacciatore with Spaghetti Squash or Palm Noodles and Roasted Kale
- Shrimp Etouffee with Okra Fries
- Shepard's Pie with Roasted Broccoli
- Beef with Chimichurri Sauce and Pan-Fried Plantain Fries

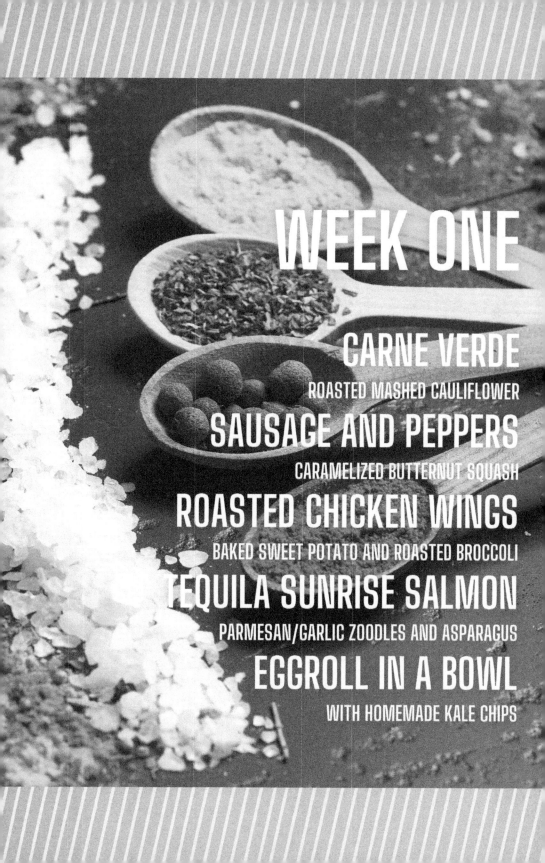

WHAT'S EATING YOU?

6 Week PREP FOR IT START UP COURSE
WEEK 1

You are at the threshold of a new "YOU" and I am thrilled to be able to provide the tools and encouragement that are needed to reach overall wellness and weight loss! The grocery list below will assist you in efficiently shopping for all of the week's necessary items. Any new essential items that have not been purchased previously are listed in the grocery list with asterisks as well. However, I encourage you to obtain these items before starting the 6-week PREP FOR IT course. You can find that full list of seasonings, condiments and sauces after the guidelines in the Resource Section of the book. Remember, we do recommend organic meats, fruits and vegetables (when able) to avoid any exposure to external hormones or pesticides.

Meat:
Chicken wings (2 pounds)
Salmon filet (enough for at least 2 6-8 ounce portions)
Ground pork (1 pound)
Ground pork (1 pound)
Pork should without bone   Chinese Chili Paste *
2 pks of Organic Italian/Cajun Chicken Sausage

Condiments, Seasoning, Oils:
Tamari or organic Soy Sauce *
Toasted Sesame Oil *
Organic Hot Wing or Mexican Sauce*
Italian Seasonings *
Chinese Chili Paste *
Verde Sauce (Hatch brand preferred)
Olive Oil *
Ghee or Organic Butter *
Organic Coconut Creme
Ground Oregano
Jar of Roasted Minced Garlic *
Black and White Sesame Seeds *
Sharachi Sauce *
Coconut Oil *
Sea Salt and Ground Pepper *
Beef Broth *
Ground Cumin, Paprika and Coffee
Onion Powder *
Almond Flour
Bag of Adobe Peppers
Coconut Aminos *

Fresh Vegetables:
1 Cauliflower Head
1 large bag slaw Shredded
1 bag fresh/frozen green beans
1 Butternut Squash
1 bag of onions (will use remainder for next week)
2 sweet potatoes
1 bag of broccoli florets
3 zucchini
2 limes
1 jalapeno
1 - red, yellow and orange bell pepper

Breakfast Foods: Eggs, organic sausage, apples

Carne Verde

Ingredients:

Pork shoulder or Pork Roast (organic) whole or cut into strips
2 tbsps. Olive, Coconut or Avocado Oil
1-2 tsp Smoked Paprika
1-2 tsp Granulated Garlic
1-2 tsp Cumin
1-2 tsp Salt
1-2 tsp Pepper
1 Tbsp Ground coffee
1-2 tsp Oregano
1-2 tsp Onion Powder
1 Tbsp Almond Flour
1 organic onion, thinly sliced
1 can green enchiladas sauce organic
1 adobe pepper
1 carton of organic beef broth (1/2 carton used for this; other 1/2 next week)

Slice onion into thin slices and set aside. Mix all dry seasonings, coffee, and almond flour together in shallow pan. Take clean dry shoulder strips and coat with seasoning mix on all sides. Pour oil into Dutch oven or porcelain pot and over medium heat, sear the meat on all sides, medium to dark brown on all sides. Remove from heat and in a slow cooker or in the Dutch oven, place 1 layer of meat in pan, then cover with onion slices. Pour half of the enchilada sauce over meat. Repeat this process with the rest of meat, onions, and sauce. Add beef broth and adobe pepper to the pan and salt and pepper. Cook on high for 1 hour and then low for 4-6 hours. When the meat is tender and breaks apart easily with fork, place on warm and serve with cauliflower mashed potatoes, sweet potatoes or cauliflower rice.

Roasted Mashed Cauliflower

If you have a heart, and for that matter, a stomach that yearns for golden mashed potatoes, but hate dealing with the carbohydrate load that follows, this recipe is an answer to prayer! Very versatile, and super easy to make! You can use frozen cauliflower to save time, but the recipe is definitely better with fresh ingredients.

Ingredients:

1 head of cauliflower
2-3 Tbsp of Ghee/butter
1-1 ½ cups of heavy cream or unsweetened almond milk
1 tsp salt
1 tsp pepper
1 tsp granulated garlic

Roasting the cauliflower in the oven first and then combining ingredients adds incredible flavor, but it certainly takes longer to prepare.

For the sake of getting in and out of the kitchen in 2 hours, start by putting the cleaned cauliflower in a microwave safe dish, and add a small amount of water to the bottom of the dish. Cover with plastic wrap and cook on high 3-4 minutes, repeating this process until the cauliflower is easily punctured with a fork. Remove and allow to cool for a few minutes (still want it to be warm). Then break up into smaller pieces.

Place the cauliflower in a food processor, add 1/2 of the milk, butter and season with salt, pepper, and granulated garlic, pulse until becomes smooth. Continue to add milk until the mixture resembles a mashed potato-like consistency. Can add additional ghee or butter to serve, and additional seasonings to taste.

Sausage, Peppers and Onions with Smothered Butternut Squash

Super easy dish to prep, and it starts to taste better the longer it sits in the fridge. When you are pinched for time, this is super quick; you prep it and place it in the oven and then you can "*fuh-ged-da-bou-dit*" and move on to something else. It really just doesn't need a lot of attention. This dish also includes your side and saves you a step in the prepping process.

Ingredients:

2 large packs of organic chicken sausage, Italian or Cajun flavors (usually 6-8 links)
1 large red, yellow, and orange pepper
1 large sweet yellow onion
3 cloves of whole garlic or 2 Tbsp of minced garlic
1 Tbsp dried Italian seasonings
1 tsp granulated garlic
1 tsp salt
1 tsp pepper
1 tsp smoked paprika
2 Tbsp organic olive oil (OO)
1 large butternut squash peeled seeded and equally cubed.

Preheat the oven to 400 degrees F. Cut the sausage into 2-inch segments and place into a disposable aluminum pan. Clean and slice peppers into ¼ inch slices and add to the aluminum pan. Thinly slice the onion and mix into the sausage and pepper mixture. In a medium mixing bowl, place the butternut squash cubes, drizzle with ½ of the OO and Italian seasoning, salt and pepper. Stir the butternut squash with tongs or a large spoon and then transfer into the aluminum pan with sausage and peppers. Add the remaining seasonings and olive oil; stir well to get all the ingredients blended well. Cover with aluminum foil; place in the oven and cook for approximately 45 minutes. Remove cover, stir and continue to cook for approximately 20 more minutes or when the peppers and onions are soft and slightly caramelized. Rustic and comforting, with no guilt!

Roasted Chicken Wings

Ingredients:

2 lbs. of organic chicken wings, trimmed
2 Tbsp granulated garlic
2 Tbsp onion powder
2 Tbsp ghee, melted
2 tsp salt
2 tsp pepper
1/4 cup of Valentina brand salsa picante hot sauce or organic buffalo sauce

Preheat oven to 400 F. Clean and dry the wings and place into a medium bowl. Pour the ghee over the chicken, hot sauce, stir well. Put bowl into the refrigerator and allow to marinate for 30-40 minutes. Remove from fridge and place on cookie sheet covered in parchment paper. Season with onion powder, garlic, salt and pepper. Cook for 45 minutes, turn all wings over and cook for an additional 30-45 minutes until the wings are golden brown and are pulling away from bone. Remove and allow to cool for 10 minutes; serve with dill/yogurt dip, non-dairy ranch, and a large salad.

Baked Sweet Potatoes

This is a staple when going through the PREP FOR IT program. Although this is considered a carbohydrate, it is extremely high in fiber and can be used with a main course or even as a snack after working out. Remember, portion control is still important and depending on the size of the sweet potato may need to cut in half to ensure staying in an appropriate daily intake.

Ingredients:

2 sweet potatoes, cleaned; remove any spots or eyes (cut out with paring knife)
Aluminum foil
Parchment paper
Cooking sheet

Preheat oven to 400 degrees.

Take clean sweet potatoes with skin on and poke holes around the potato, wrap in aluminum foil and place on parchment lined cookie sheet. Repeat with other sweet potato and place in oven, cook until able to easily puncture the potato with fork, remove and allow to cool. This can easily be eaten as a side dish, snack or used for sweet potato hash.

Roasted Broccoli

Broccoli is a great side dish for any main course. It has lots of fiber with very little carbohydrates and as a dark green vegetable, it provides lots of great vitamins.

Ingredients:

2 large broccoli heads or 1 large bag of broccoli florets (hint: go with the bag!)
1 Tbsp of dried Italian seasonings
1-2 tsp of salt
2 tsp granulated garlic
1 tsp black pepper
1/2 tsp red pepper flakes
3 Tbsp ghee or organic butter
1 Tbsp olive oil

Preheat the oven to 400 degrees F. In a mixing bowl, place the broccoli florets and pour the olive oil and melted butter over the florets; mix thoroughly to ensure that all florets are coated in the oil/butter mixture. Pour the florets into the disposable aluminum pan and then generously sprinkle with the seasonings, salt, pepper, and pepper flakes. Place in oven and cook for 45 minutes to 1 hour or until the broccoli has browned slightly and is soft when punctured with fork. This can be topped with a shredded hard cheese or can be accompanied with a feta whipped yogurt cream or just by itself!

Tequila Sunrise Salmon

Although there is no tequila in this recipe, it certainly has a tropical flair! Super easy to assemble, and the taste, well just decadent!

Ingredients:

2 pieces of thick salmon (approx. 6 x 4 inches) preferably wild caught
2 Tbsp of coconut oil
2 Tbsp of butter
Juice of 1 lime (cut 2 thin slices of lime before juicing and set aside)
1 minced 1/2 jalapeno (other half for rice)
1 tsp granulated garlic
1 Tbsp coconut cream
zest of lime
Salt/pepper to taste
Preheat oven to 375 degrees.

Clean and dry salmon filets and place in a shallow baking dish.

In the microwave or small saucepan, melt the coconut oil and butter until completely melted and add the lime juice, minced jalapeno, granulated garlic, zest and coconut cream, whisking well. Pour the mixture over the salmon; ensure that you coat all of the salmon well. Salt and pepper the tops of filets and cut the lime slices in half and place on the top of each salmon filet.

Cook at 375 degrees for approximately 10-12 minutes or until the fish flakes away, but DO NOT overcook to avoid tough or rubbery fish. Remove from oven and enjoy with coconut jalapeno cauliflower rice or roasted butternut squash.

Parmesan and Garlic Zoodles

Zucchini noodles are a great substitution for pasta, offering an increase in fiber and low carbohydrates. Sauté with ghee garlic and parmesan, and you have the perfect side dish for chicken or fish. Definitely see this recipe staying in your starting line-up!

Ingredients:

3-4 zucchini
2-3 Tbsp of Ghee/butter
1 cup of grated parmesan
1 Tbsp minced garlic
1 tsp pepper
1/2 cup unsweetened coconut or almond milk

You can make noodles using a peeling device with a noodle attachment or use the device where the zucchini is twisted into the device to make noodles, either way will work for the recipe (if unsure about the equipment or how to make the noodles refer to the Essentials video to review steps). Once noodles are done, place on a paper towel lined cookie sheet to allow to dry. In a small sauce pan, melt butter or ghee and add garlic, stirring for 1-2 minutes then add parmesan cheese and slowly add milk while stirring. When cheese is melted, add the noodles and cook on medium heat until the noodles are cooked and coated with cheese mixture. Now, simply enjoy!

Eggroll In a Bowl:

This is an incredibly simple dish to make, loaded with tons of flavor and tastes even better when it is reheated. This recipe is an absolute favorite in our kitchen.

Ingredients:

2 lbs. of organic ground meat (1 lb ground beef/1 lb ground pork)
1/4 cup of tamari
1 ½ Tbsp toasted sesame oil
1 tsp sea salt
1 tsp pepper
1 tsp Chinese chili paste
2 Tbsp coconut aminos
1 16 oz. bag of organic shredded cabbage or coleslaw with matchstick carrots

Toasted sesame seeds or dried sea weed and sesame seed sprinkles

Brown ground meat and drain. Add 1 Tbsp toasted sesame oil to heated skillet and then add bag of slaw and cook until slightly softened. Add tamari, remaining sesame oil, salt, pepper, chili paste and coconut aminos; mix well. Stir well, then remove from heat, sprinkle with sesame seeds and serve. Add additional seasonings to taste.

Kale Chips

We love kale chips, and they go with almost everything. Wait! Take that back, they go with absolutely everything! Super easy, and you can change up seasonings to achieve a different taste to the chips making the possibilities endless. It's ok to thank me later!

Ingredients:

1 large pack of kale pieces (washed and dried COMPLETELY; this is extremely important!)
1 tsp of olive oil
1 tsp of granulated garlic
1 tsp smoked paprika
1 tsp onion powder
1 tsp salt
1 tsp pepper

Preheat the oven on roast at 325 degrees F. (Cooking these at a lower temperature will dry them out, creating a crispier texture.)

Remove any tough stems from kale pieces and place the completely dried kale into a mixing bowl; sprinkle with the olive oil and then massage the leaves to coat all leaves well. Spread the leaves out onto the parchment lined baking sheet, and then sprinkle the seasonings over all of the leaves. Place in the oven and bake for approximately 30-40 minutes, checking them often to ensure they are not overcooked or burnt. Remove and can be eaten warm or even cooled. Now if you want to live on the wild side, be creative with your seasonings, and if you would love a little something to dip the chip in, consider dry ranch dressing mix in yogurt for a great snack during the day!

PLAY BY PLAY
WEEK ONE
6 Week PREP FOR IT START UP COURSE

Just as an athlete may train for a big event, you have begun to embark on a similar journey. For the athlete, there is usually a specific caloric diet and nutritional plan that will enhance workouts and promote greater performance. None of which, come easy to the athlete. It takes hard work, commitment and sacrifice. Just as it will for you.

The 6-week PREP FOR IT program provides a specific eating plan that will help you to minimize bad habits, begin proactively planning and obtain those weight loss and wellness goals you have been striving to achieve. Most athletes can reach higher levels of performance when mentored and trained by a coach. Our play-by-play steps are provided to work with you to make prepping and planning easier and more efficient. Something to keep in mind when working through each week, is realizing prepping for the week will take some time, but the ultimate goal is to get in and out of the kitchen within 2-3 hours. Now that may sound a little overwhelming and maybe even time-consuming. However, consider the following: we would spend approximately 2-3 hours watching a moving in the theater or at home, maybe getting a mani and pedi treatment at the local nail salon, or spending several hours during the day scrolling through the latest memes on social media. Keep in mind, if we can spend 2-3 hours doing these things, we should be easily able to dedicate the same amount of time to establishing proactive plans and strategies for healthy eating and weight loss.

Whether you have little to no skill in the kitchen or you are proficient enough to consider starting your own restaurant, the play-by-play instructions provide the direction to get in and out of the kitchen timely, all while cooking an amazing list of meals for the week!

Remember before you begin prepping for the next week, work through your PEER steps, figuring out what worked well, what didn't, what tasted amazing and what you could live without to begin customizing the plan moving forward. I strongly encourage writing in the margins of the recipes to allow for your own personalized taste, as you go through the program.

WHAT'S EATING YOU?

Bullet Points:

- The meals that take longer to prepare and cook should be started on first.
- ·Review the weekly menu and collect all of the ingredients, condiments, and seasonings. Sort with each individual dish/tray.
- Wash all vegetables first to expedite the prep.
- ·Clean utensils and kitchen equipment as you go to minimize the cleaning in the end.

Supplies:

Parchment Paper	Aluminum Pans (3-4)	Slow cooker
Skillet x 2	Cookie Sheets	Mixing bowls (med, large)
Prep/storage container	Spatula	Tongs x 2
Cutting knives	Cutting board	Measuring cups/spoons
Ziplock bags	Whisk or fork	

- Preheat oven 400 degrees

- Cut the pork per the recipe recommendations and season the meat, put aside. (The seasoning can be mixed at any time and store in the pantry).

- Take the washed sweet potatoes and poke with fork or small paring knife and wrap in aluminum foil. Place on parchment lined cookie sheet and put in the oven.

- Slice onions, peppers, and other veggies and put aside.

- Put olive oil into a heated Dutch oven and braise the pork pieces layering into the slow cooker with other ingredients (meat, onions, Verde sauce, meat, onion, Verde) Pour in broth and start slow cooker on high for approximately 1 hour.

- Cut sausage into 2" pieces, and place in aluminum pan. Put sliced onion, peppers, and other ingredients over sausage. Mix with tongs, cover with aluminum foil, and place in oven.

- Clean chicken wings, dry and place into a large mixing bowl with the ingredients from the recipe. Mix well with tongs and then place wings, single layer, onto a parchment lined cookie sheet. Put in the fridge at this time.

- ·Zoodle 2 zucchini, put in a small bowl and set aside.

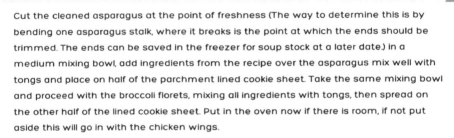

Cut the cleaned asparagus at the point of freshness (The way to determine this is by bending one asparagus stalk, where it breaks is the point at which the ends should be trimmed. The ends can be saved in the freezer for soup stock at a later date.) in a medium mixing bowl, add ingredients from the recipe over the asparagus mix well with tongs and place on half of the parchment lined cookie sheet. Take the same mixing bowl and proceed with the broccoli florets, mixing all ingredients with tongs, then spread on the other half of the lined cookie sheet. Put in the oven now if there is room, if not put aside this will go in with the chicken wings.

Clean the salmon, and placed in an aluminum pan. Salt, pepper and cover with granulated garlic. Mince the jalapeno and put aside. In a large measuring cup add all of the ingredients from the recipe. Add the jalapeno to the mixture, blend well with fork or whisk and pour over the salmon. Place a slice of lime over each piece of salmon. Set aside.

Check on sausage & pepper dish as well as the sweet potatoes. Should be ready to come out of the oven.

Start on the egg roll in a bowl recipe over the stove. Follow the recipe and when done this can be stored in prep or storage container.

Remove the sausage and peppers when the onions and peppers are caramelized (browned well) and remove sweet potatoes when able to puncture easily with fork or paring knife. Place both meals on the counter to cool.

Place the chicken wings and broccoli/asparagus into the oven. When the broccoli and asparagus are done, remove and allow to cool on countertop.

Put the salmon into the oven and allow to cook according to the recipe.

While last of food is cooking, prepare the zoodles in a skillet according to the recipe and place in a prep container. Allow to cool.

When salmon is ready (flakes easily but DO NOT overcook) then remove and allow to cool. Remove the chicken when meat is pulling away from bone.

Allow all of the meals to cool and then store in either prep or storage containers. Either throw the aluminum pans away or clean (individual preference), parchment away and clean the equipment and utensils that have not already been cleaned during prep.
·You have PREPPED now, Eat, Evaluate and get ready to Repeat!

WEEK TWO

BEEF AND BROCCOLI
WITH CAULIFLOWER RICE

HONEY MUSTARD BAKED CHICKEN
HASSELBECK POTATOES AND RATATOUILLE

KOREAN BEEF LETTUCE WRAPS
WITH ASIAN BRUSSEL SPROUT SLAW

BUFFALO CHICKEN SALAD
HOMEMADE RANCH DRESSING OVER MIXED GREENS WITH RATATOUILLE

PECAN CRUSTED TROUT
MUSHROOM PILAF CAULIFLOWER RICE AND SAUTEED GREEN BEANS

6 Week PREP FOR IT START UP COURSE
WEEK 2

You are doing it! We are moving into the second week of our 6-week prep for its series, we hope that not only were the meals very filling but delicious as well. Remember, that we are providing a grocery list for the items that you will need this week. Please check in with the essentials list located in the introduction section of the PREP for it library, as well as in the resource section of the book. Remember, if able buy organic!

Meat:
1 lb. Flank/Skirt Steak (1 strip)
1.5 lbs. or 4 Boneless/Skinless Chicken Thighs
½ Rotisserie Chicken (use other half on off days with salad
1- 1/2 lb. of ground beef and ground pork
2 Catfish or Cod Fillets (approx. 4-5 oz each)

Fresh Vegetables:
1 red onion
1-bag of cauliflower rice/1 bag pilaf cauliflower rice
Small thumb of fresh ginger
2-medium red or yellow potatoes
1-eggplant
1-small container of heirloom cherry tomatoes
3-onion (from last week's bag)
2-stalks of celery or small bunch
1-container of organic Spring Mix
1-lb clean/cut fresh green beans or kale

Condiments, Seasoning, Oils:
Honey *
Tapioca Starch *
Organic Coconut Sugar/Monk Sweetener *
Mothers® Korean Sauce *
Grey Poupon® or Organic brown mustard
Organic Ranch Mix or Dressing *
Dried chili peppers
Small bag of finely chopped pecans
Dried chili peppers
Cayenne pepper *
Dried parsley, rosemary and oregano *
1 can organic tomato paste
Olive oil mayonnaise

Breakfast Food:
**3 apples, grain-free granola organic sausage
Remaining 1/2 dozen eggs**

Slow-cooker Beef and Broccoli

Great alternative to traditional beef and broccoli with all of the great flavors, without any of the guilt! This will be on your regular rotation.

Ingredients:

1 flank or skirt steak (this can easily be doubled and put in freezer for later)
Tapioca (potato) starch approx. 1 Tbsp
1 cup of coconut sugar or 1/2 cup of monk sweetener
1 cup of tamari sauce (organic soy sauce)
1 cup water
3 dried chili peppers
2 tsp salt
2 tsp pepper
2 Tbsp minced garlic
1/4 cup of coconut aminos
1-2 large heads of broccoli
1 cup of diced scallions/green onions

If cooking in the conventional oven, preheat oven to 400 F. Can be cooked in oven or slow cooker. If cooking in slow cooker, cook on low for approximately 3-4 hours. Clean and dry beef and cut into 1–2-inch strips and place in bowl. Sprinkle beef with tapioca starch, salt and pepper; stir to completely cover all beef. Place in a 9x13 aluminum pan or in slow cooker. Chop broccoli flowers into small sizes, clean and add to the beef. Add coconut sugar, tamari, water, coconut aminos, and dried chili peppers. Cook on low for 3-4 hours in slow cooker and approximately 1 ½ -2 hours in the oven, covered with aluminum foil. Remove aluminum foil 30-40 minutes before cooking is finished. Serve over cauliflower rice.

Honey-Mustard Baked Chicken Thighs

This is a super easy recipe to throw together with your weekly prepping or even if you want to get it together during the week as well!

Ingredients:

2 lbs. of boneless, skinless chicken thighs (approx. 6-8 thighs)
2-3 tablespoons of clarified butter or ghee
1 ½ Tbsp of organic brown/spicy mustard
2 Tbsp of organic honey (can substitute manuka honey)
1 tsp salt
1 tsp cayenne pepper
1 tsp dried parsley and oregano
Preheat oven to 400 degrees.

Clean and dry chicken thighs and place in a shallow baking dish. In the microwave or small saucepan, melt the butter. Mix with the brown mustard and honey until well combined. Pour the mixture over the chicken thighs, ensure that you coat the chicken well and then season with salt, cayenne pepper, and dried herbs. Cook at 400 degrees for approximately 20-25 minutes or until the chicken is cooked through, avoiding overcooking to prevent drying out of the chicken. Remove from oven and enjoy with Hasselbeck potatoes or roasted butternut squash.

Stuffed Hasselbeck Potatoes

Potatoes are a great source of vitamins and nutrients when eaten the right way and in the right quantity. This particular recipe accompanies chicken beef or even fish really well and 1 small potato is a substantial side for any great dish.

Ingredients:

2-4 medium size organic yellow potatoes (4 if doubling the recipe)
Fresh parsley
Fresh rosemary
Organic butter or ghee
1 Tbsp fresh or jarred minced garlic
Finely shredded parmesan cheese for garnish if permitted on diet plan
1 tsp salt
1 tsp pepper

Preheat oven to 400 degrees F.

Thoroughly wash and dry potatoes. On cutting board, place the potato between 2 thin cutting boards and thinly slice the potatoes. (To prevent slicing through the potato, you can place the potato on a cutting board and then slide additional cutting boards up to each side of the potato to ensure you do not cut though the potato. For additional instructions and demonstration please refer to the Essentials 101 video for more information.)

The potatoes will be sliced almost all the way through but should be still connected approximately 1/2 inch at the bottom. Slightly separate the potatoes, avoiding pulling the potatoes apart. Place the potatoes on a parchment covered cookie sheet.

In microwave, melt butter and add parsley, rosemary, and garlic. Pour the mixture equally over the four potatoes and generously sprinkle with salt and pepper. Cook for approximately 45 minutes to 1 hour or until a fork is able to easily puncture the potato. Remove from the oven and garnish with additional parsley and parmesan if applicable.

Ratatouille

This recipe can be served over cauliflower rice as a great vegetarian main course, or in this presentation, as a very flavorful side dish that can accompany almost any poultry, beef or fish. Super easy to prepare, the superstar here is the melding of the vegetables that gives you such a comfort with every bite along with lots of vitamins and nutrients.

Ingredients:

1 large eggplant
2 zucchinis
2 yellow squash
1 sweet yellow onion
1 small container of organic cherry tomatoes (heirloom here would be amazing!)
1 Tbsp minced fresh or jarred garlic
1 Tbsp olive oil
1 Tbsp of dried Italian seasonings
1-2 tsp salt
1-2 tsp pepper
1 tsp sweet paprika (try smoked for a more Moroccan taste
1 Tbsp fresh chopped parsley
1 Tbsp fresh grated parmesan if permitted on diet plan

Preheat the oven on roast at 400 degrees F.

Cut the eggplant, zucchini, and squash into 1-1 ½ inch cubes and place in a large mixing bowl. Thinly slice the onion, separate the slices and place into the mixing bowl. Add washed and dried whole cherry tomatoes into the mixing bowl. Now add the olive oil and mix thoroughly, ensuring that all of the vegetables are coated with the olive oil. Add the garlic and seasonings to the mixing bowl and stir thoroughly; reserve 1 tsp of your salt and pepper to hit the top of the veggies before placing in the oven. Transfer the mixture to a disposable aluminum pan and then sprinkle with extra salt and pepper to your taste. (I will occasionally sprinkle the top with more of the sweet paprika as well). Place in the oven uncovered and cook for 60-80 minutes, stirring occasionally. The dish is complete when the eggplant is caramelized well (browned and yummy looking). Remove from oven and garnish with the fresh parsley and parmesan and voila, your side is done!

Korean Lettuce Wraps

Ingredients:

1/2 lb of organic ground meat and 1/2 lb of organic ground pork
1 large ripe pear or red apple
1 Tbsp toasted sesame oil (1/2 for meat and 1/2 to use with the sauce)
1 toe of fresh ginger (1 tsp)
1 Tbsp of fresh or jarred minced garlic
1 small sweet yellow onion
1 cup of matchstick carrots
1 Tbsp coconut sugar
1 Tbsp of tamari (gluten free soy sauce)
2 tsp fish sauce
1/4 cup of fermented Korean paste
1/2 cup of beef broth (more as needed to thin out sauce)
1 can of chopped water chestnuts
1 bunch fresh organic green onions for garnish
1 tsp light sesame seeds (avoid if on clean eating plans)
1 tsp of organic tomato paste
1 head of Butter leaf lettuce

Remove skin from pear or apple and finely chop or grate; put aside. Finely chop onion. Mince the ginger. In a saucepan over medium heat, put oil in pan until it coats the pain evenly and add the meat; brown evenly, seasoning with salt, pepper, and granulated garlic. Drain excess oil and add pear, onion, garlic, and ginger; stir and cook until the vegetables soften. Add salt and pepper as needed. Add the tamari, tomato paste, chili paste, sugar, remaining sesame oil and beef broth. Allow the mixture to boil and then reduce the heat to simmer, add carrots and chestnuts in and continue cooking an additional 10-15 minutes. Garnish with green onions and sesame seeds. Serve this heavenly concoction on butter leaf lettuce leaves for a scrumptious lunch or dinner.

Asian Slaw

This is an incredibly easy side dish to prepare and goes with chicken wings, hamburgers, and of course, our Korean lettuce wraps. This is such a cool contrast to the spicy wraps and complements the dish well with a crunchy edge to the dish. It definitely elevates the lettuce wraps to a whole other level!

Ingredients:

1 bag of cabbage slaw (can usually find Asian slaw mix in the produce section)
1 Tbsp sesame oil
1 tsp of rice wine vinegar
1 Tbsp almond butter or peanut butter if not on clean eating plan (optional)
1 tsp of granulated garlic
1/2 tsp ground ginger
1 Tbsp Tamari or Soy Sauce
1/2 tsp chili paste (optional as the lettuce wraps are spicy, but this does add a bit of flavor)
1 tsp onion powder
1/2 tsp pepper

Mix all wet ingredients in a bowl or large measuring cup; add spices to the mix and whisk well, until the butter is completely blended. In a separate mixing bowl, add the cleaned and dried slaw and then pour ingredients over the slaw. Using tongs, mix well, ensuring all the slaw has been coated. Serve with lettuce wraps or as a side for chicken or burgers!

Buffalo Chicken Salad (Mason Jar Salad)

Making something that is spicy, yet super easy is a double win for anyone who preps for the week. I like the fact that you simply use a rotisserie chicken as the base for the salad and all of the cooking has been done by someone else, you are simply assembling. Creating balance in prepping for the week is making sure that if there are any complex dishes to undertake, there are also some very easy ones that help alleviate longer kitchen prep times. The added flavor to this dish, well that is just a bonus!

Ingredients:

1/2 organic rotisserie chicken from local market (plain seasoning)
1-2 Tbsp paleo-friendly or organic buffalo sauce
1 tsp salt
1/4 tsp pepper (optional)
2 Tbsp finely chopped celery
1 Tbsp finely chopped red onion
1 tsp smoked paprika
1 tsp granulated garlic
1 tsp onion powder
1 Tbsp organic dry ranch mix or dressing
Boiled egg (optional)
1 Tbsp Olive oil mayonnaise or paleo-friendly mayonnaise

Remove the meat from 1/2 the rotisserie chicken and roughly chop into 1-inch cubes (nothing precise here!), Place in a medium mixing bowl. Add all ingredients and blend well. Store in the fridge for at least 1 hour, but if it's stored for at least 1 day, the flavors will have melded together. This can easily be the base for a Mason jar salad; if so, place the chicken salad into the bottom of a mason jar, add cucumbers, more thinly sliced red onions, and small heirloom tomatoes. Then add mixed greens or your favorite salad green and close the lid. It's spicy and simple!

Pecan Crusted Trout

Ingredients:
2 fresh trout or white fish filets
1 cup of Pork rind Panko Crumbs
1 cup of minced pecans (organic preferred)
1 tsp fresh or dried minced rosemary
1 tsp fresh or dried minced oregano
3-4 Tbsp of almond flour (1 Tbsp to be used in the pecan mixture)
1 organic egg, lightly beaten
1-2 tsp of salt
1-2 tsp of pepper
1 Tsp granulated garlic
3 Tbsp ghee (clarified butter 1 ½ to use for cooking and 1 ½ to drizzle on cooked fish)
1 Tbsp fresh parsley

Place the almond flour in a shallow dish and season with salt, pepper, and granulated garlic; then thoroughly mix flour with a fork. In a shallow bowl, slightly whisk 1 egg and sprinkle with salt and pepper. In 3rd shallow dish, mix remaining almond flour, minced pecans, rosemary, and oregano thoroughly, seasoning again with salt pepper and granulated garlic. This part can get messy, but it is extremely worth it. Dredge, (pull the filet through the flour and then flip over and coat the opposite site) shaking off any excess. Then dredge the filet through the egg mixture, ensuring that it is coated well. Allow the excess to fall back into the egg mixture. Then dredge this filet into the pecan mixture and push the ingredients down onto the filet, making sure it covers all parts of the fish. Place on a clean plate and heat your frying pan or griddle to medium heat.

Add 1 ½ of the ghee to the pan and allow it to melt and coat the entire pan. You can substitute olive oil here, but it will not be as decadent! When the ghee is melted (do not let this brown too much or it will burn and can cause the fish to taste burnt). Place the filets into the pan and press down with a spatula. DO NOT move the filets, allowing them to cook on the first side for at least 3-5 minutes. Carefully release the filet from the pan with the spatula and flip over to the uncooked side and cook for an additional 2- 4 minutes. Remove filets and place on a clean plate. Wipe the pan with a clean paper towel and then add the remaining ghee with the fresh parsley, stirring for about 2-3 minutes. Drizzle this mixture over the filets prior to serving. Super easy prep with tons of flavor.

Cauliflower Rice Pilaf with Fresh Cremini Mushrooms

Ingredients:

1 bag of frozen cauliflower rice (or rice one fresh cauliflower; however, this will need to be cooked)
1 Tbsp finely chopped parsley
1 Tbsp ghee or organic butter
1-1 ½ cups of cremini or Porcini mushrooms, finely sliced.
1 tsp salt
1 tsp pepper
1 tsp granulated garlic

In a medium saucepan, heat up the ghee or butter until completely melted; add onions and mushrooms and cook on medium heat until soft and onion is translucent. Stirring occasionally, increase heat to medium high and add the bag of cauliflower rice, salt, pepper, and granulated garlic. Cook for approximately 7-8 minutes on high to ensure that additional water is cooked off and you have a great rice consistency. Garnish with parsley or shredded parmesan. Great served with fish or chicken.

Sauté Green Beans

Green beans are typically the only "green" vegetables many individuals will consider eating when it comes to healthy options. However, with a few seasonings, fresh ingredients, and the right cooking method, I am confident this will be a "go to" recipe for you in the future!

Ingredients:

1 bag or 1 lb of loose fresh green beans
1 Tbsp of Ghee/butter
1 onion, thinly sliced
1 Tbsp minced garlic
1 small piece of Tasso (spicy ham), cubed
1/4 cup of dry cooking sherry
1 tsp salt
1 tsp pepper
1 tsp granulated garlic

In a medium saucepan heat up the ghee or butter until completely melted; add cubed Tasso and cook until ends are slightly brown. Then add onions and pepper. Cook until the onions are just slightly translucent, add the garlic and cook an additional 1-2 minutes. Add sherry or water and deglaze the pot. Add cleaned green beans and if needed, add additional water, additional seasonings, cover and simmer for approximately 20-25 minutes, stirring occasionally. Green beans should be slightly al dente (firm) and still be bright green in color. Remove from stove top and allow to cool; place in prepared container. Super easy and super yummy!

PLAY BY PLAY
WEEK TWO

6 Week PREP FOR IT START UP COURSE

Working through the play-by-play for week one you have likely identified the workflow of your kitchen, what works great and then what presents a few challenges. Make sure before beginning week two, that you have worked through the PEER steps (Prep, Eat, Evaluate, Repeat) to provide you with the greatest chance for success.

Bullet Points:

- The meals that take longer to prepare and cook should be started on first.
- Review the weekly menu and collect all of the ingredients, condiments, and seasonings. Sort with each individual dish/tray.
- Wash all vegetables first to expedite the prep.
- Clean utensils and kitchen equipment as you go to minimize the cleaning in the end.

Supplies:

Parchment Paper	Aluminum Pans (3-4)	Slow cooker
Skillet x 2	Cookie Sheets	Mixing bowls (med, large)
Prep/storage container	Spatula	Tongs x 2
Cutting knives	Cutting board	Measuring cups/spoons
Ziplock bags	Whisk or fork	

- Preheat oven 400 degrees

- Cut the beef into strips according to the recipe and place in a ziplock bag. Coat with the starch and put into the fridge.

- Cut all veggies according to the different recipes and put aside. This should include, broccoli, ratatouille vegetables, mushrooms and the potatoes according to the recipe and put aside in designated trays.

- Clean the chicken thighs, dry and place into aluminum pan. Mix the seasonings for the honey mustard chicken and pour over the chicken. Cover with foil and place in the fridge for now.

- Place all vegetable for the ratatouille into an aluminum pan, coat with olive oil, all seasonings and add salt, pepper and granulated garlic. Mix with tongs and cover with aluminum foil and put into the oven. Set a timer.

WHAT'S EATING YOU?

- Take the beef out of the fridge and place in the slow cooker. Add all the ingredients from the recipe, then add the broccoli, mix well with tongs and cover. Start the slow cooker on high for approximately 1 hour.

- Melt the butter in a large mixing cup and add the seasonings blending well. Place the potatoes in an aluminum pan and pour the mixture over the potatoes. Add salt, pepper and parsley and put in the oven.

- Bring all ingredients for the Korean wraps to the oven, including the chopped pear and onion. (consider chopping the pear just before cooking to avoid browning of the fruit.) Brown the ground meat in a heated and oiled skillet according to the recipe and cook. When complete allow to cool and place in a prep or storage container. The lettuce should be washed already and allowed to dry store in sealed container in fridge. Mix up the Asian slaw and place in covered container in the fridge.

- Check the ratatouille, mixing with the tongs. Leave uncovered and cook until brown on the edges and able to insert fork easily into the veggies.

- Cut the rotisserie chicken breast and 1 leg and thigh off and remove meat from bone. Then cube or shred the chicken. Place the chicken pieces into a large mixing bowl, add all of the ingredients following the recipe and mix well. This can be packed in a mason jar with the salad fixings placed on top. This makes storage and serving easy. Put in the fridge.

- When the ratatouille is done remove from oven and allow to cool and then place in prep or storage container. Take the chicken out of the fridge and place in the oven and set the timer. Check the beef and broccoli and lower the temperature at this time.

- Clean the trout or catfish and dry. Set up the dredging station, season the fish, then dredge the filets. Heat the skillet and add ghee or butter and cook the trout, following the recipe. Allow to cool and place in a prep or storage container.

- Cook the onions and mushroom slices in a heated skillet with olive oil and add the cauliflower rice and cook according to the recipe. When cooked transfer to a prep or storage container trout can be placed over the rice or on the side to save space.

- Remove the potatoes and chicken when done. Cool and then place in appropriate prep or storage container. When beef and broccoli done, place in a prep or storage container allow to cool prior to transferring into the fridge. Throw away all disposable equipment, clean skillets, and utensils.

WEEK THREE

EVERYTHING BAGEL COD
BAKED SWEET POTATO/CREAMY SPINACH

CHICKEN ENCHILADAS & FIXINS
WITH TURMERIC LIME BROCCOLI RICE

BACON MUSHROOM BURGER
WITH ZUCCHINI PARMESAN FRIES

SMOTHERED PORKCHOPS, ONIONS, & MUSHROOMS
SWEET POTATO MASH

COMBINATION FRIED RICE
WITH SAUTEED ASIAN CABBAGE

WHAT'S EATING YOU?

6 Week PREP FOR IT START UP COURSE
WEEK 3

You are starting to get your groove on! We are reaching the halfway mark going into the third week of our 6-week PREP FOR IT series, and I hope your starting to see some great results while enjoying some delicious dishes in the process. Remember, that we are providing a grocery list for the items that you will need this week with any essentials not already purchased. Please check in with the essentials list to ensure you are stocked and ready for the week! Go organic!

Meat:
2-large pc of trout or cod
6-organic chicken breast (approx 2-3 lbs)
1-lb organic ground beef
2-3 organic pork chops (1/2 inch to ¾ thick)
1-skirt steak
½-pound fresh frozen shrimp peeled
1 pound bacon (1/2 for burger)
1 rotisserie chicken

Fresh Vegetables:
4-sweet potatoes
1 bunch fresh parsley
3-cauliflower head or 3 bags of cauliflower rice
1-lime
Cilantro (optional)
3-zucchini
1 small bag frozen peas (store rest for week 6)
2 organic carrots
1-small cabbage head
5 onions (may have some left from week 1 or get new bag)
1/2 pound of porcini or cremini mushrooms
1 avocado

Condiments, Seasoning, Oils:
1 can Red Enchilada Sauce
Everything bagel seasoning mix *
Coconut flour, fine *
Bay leaves *
Chipotle pepper *
Organic Cooking Sherry * (optional)
Ground Turmeric
fresh ginger (leftover last week or ground)
Fish Sauce *
1 bag shredded organic Mexican cheese (optional)
1 container organic sour cream or almond milk sour cream
1 pk. almond tortillas (Siete® preferred)

Breakfast food: protein shakes, eggs, sausage

Everything Bagel Cod Filets

Ingredients:

2 large fresh cod, trout or white fish filets
3 heaping Tbsp of everything bagel seasoning (online or specialty store)
3 Tbsp of coconut flour (1 Tbsp to be used in the pecan mixture)
1 organic egg, lightly beaten
1 tsp salt for wash (1/2 for egg mixture 1/2 for crust seasoning)
2 tsp each of sea salt and pepper
1 tsp granulated garlic
3 Tbsp ghee (clarified butter 1 ½ to use for cooking and 1 ½ to drizzle on cooked fish)
1 Tbsp fresh parsley

Place the coconut flour in a shallow dish and season with salt, pepper and granulated garlic; then thoroughly mix flour with a fork. In a shallow bowl, slightly whisk 1 egg and sprinkle with salt and pepper. In 3rd shallow dish, mix remaining coconut flour with the everything bagel seasonings. Then thoroughly season the filets with salt/pepper and granulated garlic. This part can get messy, but it is extremely worth it. This is a 3-coat process that when placed in the flour first, then the egg, will allow the 3rd mixture to adhere to the fish without falling off during the cooking process.

Dredge (pull the filet through the flour and then flip over and coat the opposite site) shaking off any excess. Then dredge the filet through the egg mixture; ensure that it is coated well. Allow the excess to fall back into the egg mixture. Dredge this filet into the everything bagel mixture and push the ingredients down onto the filet, making sure it covers all parts of the fish. Place on a clean plate and repeat with second filet. Heat your frying pan or griddle to medium heat. Add 1 ½ of the ghee to the pan and allow it to melt and coat the entire pan. You can substitute olive oil here, but it will not be as decadent! When the ghee is melted, (do not let this brown too much as it will burn and can cause the fish to taste burnt) place the filets into the pan and press down with a spatula. DO NOT move the filets, allowing them to cook on the first side for at least 3-5 minutes. Carefully release the filet from the pan with the spatula and flip over to the uncooked side and cook for an additional 2- 4 minutes. Remove filets and place on a clean plate. Wipe the pan with a clean paper towel and then add the remaining ghee with the fresh parsley and stir for about 2-3 minutes. Drizzle this mixture over the filets prior to serving. Super easy prep with tons of flavor.

Baked Sweet Potatoes

Ingredients:

2 sweet potatoes, cleaned and remove any spots or eyes (cut out with paring knife)
Aluminum foil
Parchment paper
Cooking sheet

Preheat oven to 400 degrees. Take clean sweet potatoes with skin on and poke holes around the potato, wrap in aluminum foil, and place on parchment lined cookie sheet. Repeat with other sweet potato and place in oven, cook until able to easily puncture the potato with fork, remove and allow to cool.

Creamy Guilt-Free Spinach

Creamy spinach is a great way to get those dark green leafy veggies into your eating plan, and what better way than making a nice creamy, and yes, healthy cream sauce to compliment this veggie. You can use either fresh or frozen spinach, just make sure to get any excess water out of the frozen spinach before preparing.

Ingredients:

1 large bag of baby spinach leaves (baby leaves have stems that do not need to be removed.)
1 container of almond milk cream cheese (plain preferred)
1 Tbsp of Ghee or butter
1 Tbsp minced garlic
1/2 cup grated parmesan cheese
1 tsp salt and 1 tsp pepper
1 Tbsp Dijon mustard
1 shallot
1 Tbsp coconut flour or very fine almond flour
1 cup of chicken or bone broth
Organic bacon bits for garnish (optional)

In a medium skillet, melt the ghee and then add the flour, stirring continuously over low to medium heat until completely blended. Continue cooking for approximately 3-4 minutes, stirring constantly. Stir in shallots, salt, and pepper and continue to cook for approximately 2-3 minutes, stirring or whisking. Add the garlic, cream cheese, and mustard, cooking an additional 1-2 minute until the cheese is completely blended. Slowly add the chicken broth while stirring, then add the parmesan cheese. Reduce the heat, adding the spinach to the mixture. Consider covering the skillet for 1 minute; then remove the cover and stir the mixture until well blended and the spinach is wilted.

Chicken Enchilada Taco Bowl

I love this recipe! It is super easy, has lots of flavor, and can be used for family get-togethers without a big fuss. Add tortillas for heartier meal.

Ingredients:

Organic chicken thighs or chicken breast (approx. 2-3 lbs.)
1 onion
1 tsp minced garlic
1 tsp paprika
1 tsp salt
1 tsp pepper
1 tsp cumin
1 tsp ground oregano
1 tsp onion powder
2 bay leaves
1 chipotle pepper, dried
1 can red enchilada sauce (preferably organic)
Bay leaf
Avocado (to serve)
Cilantro
Sour cream
1 lime (wedges for serving)
1 container organic Mexican cheese (optional)
Almond flour tortilla or cauliflower rice (accompany with meal)

Clean and dry chicken. Mix all dry ingredients in a bowl, then coat all chicken with the seasoning and place in slower cooker. Slice the onions into thin slices and place over the chicken; pour the enchilada sauce over the chicken and onions. Add bay leaves, and dried pepper; cover and cook on low for 4-6 hours. Check chicken at 4 hours and using a fork, pull all chicken pieces apart continue to cook on low for another hour. Serve with cilantro, organic sour cream, lime wedges, over cauliflower rice or on grain-free soft tacos.

Turmeric, Cilantro and Lime Broccoli Rice

This is a fabulous side dish that brings great flavor and balance to the chicken enchiladas, Carne Verde, or even the barbacoa beef. Extremely easy to make and reheats well!

Ingredients:

1-bag of frozen broccoli rice
1/2 chopped onion
1 lime zested and juiced
1 Tbsp minced garlic
1 Tbsp finely chopped Cilantro
1 Tbsp Coconut Oil
1 tsp turmeric
1 tsp salt
1 tsp pepper
1 tsp onion powder

In a medium saucepan, heat up the oil until completely melted; add onions, cook on medium heat until soft and onion is translucent. Add salt and pepper, stirring occasionally. Increase heat to medium high and add the bag of broccoli rice and remaining seasonings. Cook for approximately 5-7 minutes on med/high to ensure that additional water is cooked off and you have a great rice consistency. Add the lime juice, zest and stir thoroughly. Garnish with cilantro; store in prep container. This partners well with the chicken enchiladas or even the Carne Verde.

Bacon and Mushroom Burgers

Eat these great burgers solo or between 2 Portobello or no grain hamburger buns for a hearty hamburger option! It makes 4 – 1/2 lb burgers; you can easily double the recipe here and freeze individual patties for later!

Ingredients:

2 lbs. of organic ground meat (cannot stress this enough grass-fed, no antibiotics will make a world of difference here)
1 tablespoon olive oil
1 medium onion, finely minced
Organic bacon, thickly cut from butcher and then cut into small cubes
1 tablespoon of minced garlic
Fresh porcini mushrooms, minced
1-2 tsp kosher salt
1 tsp of coarse black pepper

Heat olive oil in a shallow skillet on medium heat; add bacon cubes, stirring occasionally to avoid sticking. When bacon is lightly brown, add onions and mushrooms, cooking for 10-12 minutes and then add the garlic; continue to brown until completely cooked. You can 1/2 tsp salt and pepper here, but we will add the seasoning for the burgers when we add mixture to ground meat.

Once the mixture is cooked, remove from heat and allow to cool thoroughly. Put the ground meat into a medium mixing bowl and add the bacon/mushroom mixture, salt, and pepper. Combine ingredients, but do not over-mix here because it will make the burgers tough. Divide the meat into 2 equal balls and then mold into hamburger patties approximately 1-1 ¼ inch thick. Coat skillet with olive oil and heat a griddle or a large shallow skillet on medium high heat. Place the hamburger patties onto the griddle; press slightly with a spatula to sear the patty and then flip the patties after cooking on one side for approximately 5 minutes and continue cooking for approximately 5-7 minutes, pressing the patties slightly to ensure a good sear. You can cook these to your liking, depending on how seared you would like your burgers.

Zucchini Fries with Parmesan

Great substitution to conventional fries! Super easy to complete and can be eaten as a side dish or even a snack.

Ingredients:

3 zucchinis, cut into 1/2 inch sticks
1 cup Pork rind panko crumbs
1 cup grated parmesan cheese
1 tsp granulated garlic
1 dash of buffalo sauce or tabasco sauce
2 eggs, slightly beaten in shallow bowl
1/2 tsp salt
1/2 tsp pepper
Organic ranch dressing for dipping (optional)

Preheat oven to 425 degrees. In a shallow dish, lightly beat the eggs, adding 2 dashes of buffalo sauce or tabasco sauce. In a separate shallow dish, blend panko crumbs and parmesan cheese; add seasonings, blending well. Dredge the zucchini fries into the egg mixture and mix well in the cheese and panko mixture; place in a single layer on a parchment lined baking sheet. Bake approximately 25-30 minutes, rotating the pan midway through baking; turn the fries over if needed until crispy brown. Great side for our bacon burger or even chicken wings!

Smothered Pork Chops with Mushrooms and Onions

It's Southern comfort without all the guilt, or weight! Great hearty meal that not only tastes great out of the oven, but when reheated and able to sit in the fridge for a few days, has even better flavor! Just an all-around great dish.

Ingredients:

2-3-organic pork chops (approx. 3/4 to 1-inch-thick, bone in)
2 medium sweet yellow onions
1 cup of fresh sliced porcini mushrooms
1 Tbsp minced garlic or 2 cloves of minced fresh garlic
1/2 cup of organic red wine or sherry (optional)
1-1½ cups of beef broth
1Tbsp Granulated garlic
1tsp onion powder
1 tsp dried oregano
2 Tbsp olive oil
1 Tbsp butter or ghee
Salt and pepper to taste
1 Tbsp sifted almond flour

Preheat the oven at 400 degrees. Finely slice the onions and mushrooms and set aside. On a flat cookie sheet, season chops with salt, pepper, onion powder, and granulated garlic, then dust pork chops.

Heat a Dutch pot and brown the pork chops in 1 Tbsp olive oil and 1 Tbsp butter, approximately 5-7 minutes on each side. Put on separate plate. In the reserved oil, add the onions and mushrooms and cook until the onions are soft and cooked down; add remaining seasonings and salt/pepper to taste. Add the sherry (optional) and deglaze the pot, stirring to remove any debris from the pot. Then add 1 cup of beef broth until combined and a gravy consistency is obtained. Place the pork chops in an aluminum pan and pour the gravy over the meat; bake in the oven at 400 degrees F for approximately 40-50 minutes or until the meat pulls away from bone. Serve over cauliflower rice or sweet potato mash and enjoy!

Savory Sweet Potato Mash

Such a hearty, savory side dish with plenty of fiber and flavor to boot! If you are striving to continue eating healthy during the holidays, this is a great substitution for the traditional sweet potato dish.

Ingredients:

2 sweet potatoes, cleaned and baked
1/2 cup of unflavored almond milk or organic cream cheese
1 Tbsp Honey
2 Tbsp ghee or organic butter melted
1/4 tsp organic vanilla
1 Tbsp minced garlic
1 bunch green onions
1 Tbsp of fresh minced/finely chopped parsley
1/2 tsp salt
1/2 tsp pepper

Remove the potato skins from the baked sweet potatoes and discard. Place the sweet potato flesh into a mixing bowl and mash with a potato masher or hand-mixer on lowest setting. Add the green onions and parsley; continue to blend and add cream cheese, honey, butter, vanilla and salt and pepper to taste.

Combination Fried Rice (Cauliflower Rice)

Ingredients:

1 lb of skirt steak, cut into 1/2 inch slices with the grain
1 Tbsp of tapioca flour
1/2-1 lb of medium size white shrimp (wild preferred)
1 lb of cooked chicken, cubed (use 1/2 of a rotisserie chicken; super easy!)
2 Tbsp of toasted sesame oil (1 Tbsp for cooking, 1 Tbsp to garnish with after cooking)
3 organic carrots cut into small 1/8- inch cubes
1 large onion, finely diced
2 tsp of minced garlic
1 tsp of freshly grated ginger
1/2 cup of tamari (non-soy soy sauce, I know an oxymoron!)
2 Tbsp of fish sauce
1-2 tsp of Chinese chili sauce (with the green lid, seriously hot so season to taste, but beware!)
1 bunch of green onions, sliced
2 cups of cauliflower rice
1 tsp of toasted sesame seeds (optional)

Once the skirt steak is cut, place in a large ziplock bag, sprinkle the tapioca starch on the meat, close the bag and shake to evenly coat the meat. In a large skillet, heat olive oil and 1 tablespoon of sesame oil on medium heat; add the meat, stir to prevent sticking and brown thoroughly. Remove from heat and place on a dish. Add shrimp to the olive and cook shrimp, stirring until pink, but do not overcook; we will add this back in a bit. Add the 1/2 tablespoon of olive oil in pan, add onions and carrots; stir occasionally and brown for approximately 7-10 minutes. Add garlic and ginger and cook an additional 2 minutes. Add the cauliflower, turn up the heat to keep the cauliflower drier and cook for about 5-7 minutes, stirring continuously; now add the tamari, chili and fish sauce, chicken, shrimp and beef combined thoroughly. Add green onions and cook for an additional 5 minutes. Garnish with additional green onions and sesame seeds. Get creative and add mushrooms, or even organic bacon cubes to kick it up a notch!

Asian Fried Cabbage

When you are looking for an easy side dish that pairs with anything and is full of flavor, this will be your new favorite!

Ingredients:

2 bags of organic slaw mix (red and green cabbage)
1/4 cup of coconut sugar
1 Tbsp toasted sesame oil
1/2 cup of ghee or butter
1 Tbsp tamari
1/2 tsp Chinese red chili pepper sauce

Heat butter and sesame oil until butter is melted; add the coconut sugar until dissolved and add tamari and red chili sauce. Cook and stir for an additional 5 minutes. Add both bags of slaw, stirring to allow ingredients to cook down. Salt and lightly pepper to taste and allow to cook for approximately 10-15 minutes or until thoroughly wilted. Grate fresh ginger, stir and remove from heat; this is awesome with beef and broccoli or with honey orange chicken.

WHAT'S EATING YOU?

PLAY BY PLAY
WEEK THREE
6 Week PREP FOR IT START UP COURSE

Halfway through the PREP FOR IT course and chances are this week you will feel more confident in your prepping skills and have started to develop a rhythm. Keep it up! Make sure before beginning this week that you have worked through the PEER steps (Prep, Eat, Evaluate, Repeat) to provide you with the greatest chance for success.

Bullet Points:
- The meals that take longer to prepare and cook should be started on first.
- Review the weekly menu and collect all of the ingredients, condiments, and seasonings. Sort with each individual dish/tray.
- Wash all vegetables first to expedite the prep.
- Clean utensils and kitchen equipment as you go to minimize the cleaning in the end.

Supplies:

Parchment Paper	Aluminum Pans (3-4)	Slow cooker
Skillet x 2	Cookie Sheets	Mixing bowls (med, large)
Prep/storage container	Spatula	Tongs x 2
Cutting knives	Cutting board (plastic/wood)	Measuring cups/spoons
Ziplock bags	Whisk or fork	Timer

- Preheat oven 400 degrees

- Take cleaned sweet potatoes poke holes in them with paring knife or fork and wrap in foil placing them on parchment lined cookie sheet or aluminum pan.

- Cut all veggies according to the different recipes and put aside. This should include, the onions, mushrooms, carrots and zucchini. Chop the onions for the Bacon burger and the combination fried rice and put aside in designated trays.

- In the slow cooker layer chicken breast, onions, and red enchilada sauce. Cover and cook according to the recipe.

- Season the porkchops and in a heated Dutch oven braise the chops in olive oil according to the recipe and then place the braised chops in the aluminum pan. Deglaze the pain according to the recipe and add the onions and mushrooms, then the broth as instructed. Pour the mixture over the braised chops, season with salt and pepper. Cover with foil and put in the oven. Set the timer according to the recipe.

- Cook the onions, bacon, and mushrooms for the bacoburgers in a skillet and when browned put in a bowl and set aside.
- In the next skillet, cook the veggies for the combination fried rice, following the recipe. When complete put the meal in a prep or storage container and allow to cool.
- In a large mixing bowl mix the zucchini fries with olive oil, seasonings and then place in a single layer on ½ of the parchment lined cookie sheet. Sprinkle generously with parmesan or asiago cheese. Put the cleaned green beans into the same mixing boil and oil and seasonings and stir well with tongs. Place on the other ½ of the parchment lined cookie sheet, and put in the oven.
- Mix the ground meat, seasonings, and the cooled onions/bacon/mushroom mixture together (do not over mix here) in the same mixing bowl and make large patties. place the patties on a hot skillet and cook according to the recipe. Flip and continue to cook until done and transfer to a napkin lined plate to drain off excess fat. Then store in a prep or storage container.
- Check the items in the oven, turning the zucchini fries
- Set up the dredging station for the cod, season the cleaned, dry fish and in a heated skillet cook the fish in olive oil according to the recipe, when done transfer to the prep or storage container and allow to cool.
- Make the lime turmeric cauliflower rice in the skillet according to the recipe and when done transfer to the prep or storage container allowing to cool.
- Once the sweet potatoes are soft and can easily be poked with fork or paring knife remove from oven and allow to cool on countertop. Once cooled use 2 of the sweet potatoes for the sweet potato mashed recipe combining ingredients and then store in prep or storage containers.
- When zucchini fries are brow and soft/caramelized and green beans are soft remove and allow to cool on the countertop. Once cooled transfer into storage or prep containers.
- When pork chops are tender and pull away from the bone remove them from oven and allow to cool before storing.
- When chicken can be pulled apart with 2 forks turn the slow cooker down or off and shred the chicken and place into a storage or prep container.
- Throw away all disposable equipment, clean skillets, and utensils.

WEEK FOUR

CHICKEN SHAWARMA
TURMERIC/PINENUT RICE WITH CUCUMBER SALAD

BEST MEATLOAF EVER
ROASTED YELLOW BEETS AND MASHED CAULIFLOWER

CHICKEN PHO
ROASTED BROCCOLI

MISO TUNA BOWL
WITH CARROTS RIBBONS, AND FRIED RICE

PIZZA FRITTATA
WITH SWEET POTATO FRIES

WHAT'S EATING YOU?

6 Week PREP FOR IT START UP COURSE
WEEK 4

Prep, Eat, Evaluate, and Repeat! Starting week 4 of the PREP FOR IT 6-week start-up course and you should see a routine develop with your prepping process. Finding your groove is what makes PREP FOR IT successful for so many individuals. I trust the meals have been fun to prepare, and you continue to see some positive momentum for your weight loss and wellness journey. Now grab the grocery list for this week and let's go! We have added some additional essentials but you should still have plenty of seasonings for the 6-week program. As always, go organic.

Meat:
6-organic chicken breast
2-lb organic ground beef
1/2-lb organic Italian sausage (loose)
(leftover bacon from last week)
2 tuna steaks
1 dozen eggs (meatloaf and frittata)
1 pk organic pepperoni slices

Fresh Vegetables:
1-cauliflower head or cauliflower rice
4-yellow beets
1-bag of broccoli florets
1-small bag matchstick carrots (save half for next week)
1 cucumber
1 small bag of Asian slaw
1 avocado
1 lime
2 onions (grab another bag if needed)
2 sweet potatoes
1 pound okra or cut fresh green beans
2 whole carrots (ideal purple and yellow)
Large Handful of porcini mushrooms
Small bag baby spinach

Condiments, Seasoning, Oils:
Ground Cinnamon *
Dry Miso Soup mix (organic) *
Ground cloves *
(Organic Tomato Paste * (2 cans)
Bragg's Apple Cider Vinegar w/ginger & sesame
Fresh mung sprouts (optional)
1 whole nutmeg
Ground sumac (specialty store or online)
Cilantro (optional)
Jalapeno (optional)
Organic ketchup
1 container of Ocean's Halo®Pho Broth
1 pk nuPasta®Konjac Angel Hair
1 pk Epic®organic bacon bits
Balsalmic Vinegar *
½ cup pine nut
½ cup sliced almonds
Mozzarella shredded or buffalo
Sarachi sauce
Bunch of green onions

Breakfast foods: Repeat week 1

Chicken Shawarma

This is a super easy recipe that produces tons of flavor and lets your taste buds venture out into some exotic cuisines. (Your friends will rave over this one!)

Ingredients:

1 lb. of boneless, skinless chicken breast (for this recipe, but approx. 6 breasts will use 3 for pho)
2 tsp ground cumin
1/2 tsp ground chili powder
1 tsp sweet paprika
1 tsp granulated garlic
1/2 to 1 tsp sea salt
1/2 to 1 tsp cayenne pepper
1/2 tsp ground turmeric
1/2 tsp cinnamon (Saigon preferred)
Approx. 1/8 tsp of ground cloves
3/4 cup of water
1/4 cup of olive oil
1/4 cup of coconut oil

Mix all dry seasonings in a bowl and put aside. Place all clean chicken breasts into slow cooker and cover with water; cook on low for 2-3 hours. Allow to cool slightly, then cut into 1/2 inch slices against the grain. (Put 1/2 aside for our pho recipe). In a large Dutch oven or porcelain coated frying pan, heat the olive and coconut oil. When hot, add chicken slices; avoid overlapping pieces. Sprinkle 1/2 of the dry seasoning mixture onto the chicken (be generous here!) and avoid stirring for 2-3 minutes, if oil is absorbing, add a little more olive oil, turn the chicken and sprinkle the remaining seasoning onto the chicken, cooking for 2-3 minutes. Ready to serve! Great with rice or even Cucumber/Yogurt salad!

Greek Yogurt Cucumber Salad

Super easy salad to assemble and goes great with our Chicken Shawarma bowl. This also makes a great entertainment salad; so much potential, so full of flavor!

Ingredients:

1 English cucumber, cubed
1 container organic, plain yogurt or almond milk
1 Tbsp of dried or fresh dill
1 small can sliced black olives (optional)
1 red onion, quartered then sliced thin
1 cup of small organic heirloom tomatoes
1 cup of organic feta cheese
1 tsp minced garlic
1 fresh lemon, zested and juiced
1/4 cup of olive oil
1 tsp dried oregano
1 Tbsp honey
Salt and pepper to taste

Whisk all seasonings and wet ingredients together in a large measuring cup or mixing bowl and put aside. Cut the cucumbers, onions, and half the cherry tomatoes; place in a mixing bowl and blend together. Pour the dressing over the salad and mix well. This can be served immediately, but tastes even better after sitting in the fridge for a day!

Best Meatloaf Ever!

Meat loaf, we grew up with this dinner staple and likely, it was a hum-drum meal. Well, no more! The ingredients in this recipe bring meatloaf to another level, and it is sure to bring the family coming back for more!

Ingredients:

2 Medium Carrots finely chopped
1-2 Tbsp olive oil
1-1½ c. of chopped porcini mushrooms
1/2 cup of dry sherry or white wine
1/2 lb of organic Italian sausage (loose)
1-2 tsp salt/1-2 tsp pepper
2 Tbsp Pork rind Panko Crumbs
1 tsp onion powder
Organic ketchup (1 Tbsp)

1 Medium onion, finely chop
2 tsp minced roasted garlic
2 Tbsp tomato paste
2 lbs of organic ground beef
1 Tbsp Dried Italian Seasoning
1 large egg
1 tsp garlic powder
1/2 tsp cayenne pepper
4 pc bacon, cut in half

Preheat oven to 375 degrees. In a medium pot, sauté chopped carrots and onions until translucent, approximately 8-10 minutes; season with some of the salt and pepper, then add chopped mushrooms and cook for an additional 5-10 minutes, stirring occasionally. Add minced garlic and stir constantly for approximately 2-3 minutes, then add tomato paste and continue to stir for another 5 minutes; add sherry and deglaze the pan, then cook on low heat until the mixture is a medium to dark red color. Set aside and allow to cool.

In a large mixing bowl, add 2 pounds of organic beef and 1 pound of organic Italian sausage (loose). Then add the cooked mixture and the remaining ingredients. Combine the ingredients with your hands (this is the fun part) be careful not to over mix, but thoroughly combine. When completed, place in a disposable loaf pan and mold it with the middle higher and the sides of the loaf lower around the edges. Pour the additional ketchup on top and place the uncooked pieces of bacon on the top of the loaf all the way over the top of it. Cook on the middle rack (may want to put a drip pan under the loaf pan to ensure it does not drip over the edge when the meat cooks down) and cook for approximately 45 minutes to 1 hour. The loaf is done when the internal temperature reaches 165 degrees. Remove from the oven and allow to cool. Cut into thick slices then enjoy

Roasted Yellow Beets

This side dish pairs well with our meatloaf or even a rotisserie chicken. It is comforting, warm, with plenty of flavor. If beets are typically not your thing, at least give this recipe a try. You may be surprised that this is not your Mama's beets!

Ingredients:

3-4 yellow beets, cleaned and peeled
1 Tbsp Olive or Avocado Oil
1 tsp dried thyme
1 tsp salt
1 tsp pepper
1 tsp granulated garlic

Dressing:

1 Tbsp balsamic vinegar
1 Tbsp olive oil
1/2 tsp salt
1 Tbsp honey
Preheat oven to 400 degrees.

Whisk the dressing ingredients together in a large measuring cup and put aside. Cut the peeled beets and cube into the same size cubes and put in a mixing bowl. Add olive oil, stirring and then add the dry ingredients and mix well. Place on a parchment lined baking sheet and place in the oven, roasting for approximately 25-30 minutes. When the beets can be easily punctured with a fork, remove from oven and in the same mixing bowl, put the beets back in and stir in the balsamic dressing. Put back on the parchment lined baking sheet and put back into the oven for approximately 10 minutes, allowing the liquid to caramelize. Remove and allow to cool.

Roasted Mashed Cauliflower

If you have a heart, and for that matter, a stomach that yearns for golden mashed potatoes, but hate dealing with the carbohydrate load that follows, this recipe is an answer to prayer! Very versatile, and super easy to make! You can use frozen cauliflower to save time, but the recipe is definitely better with fresh ingredients.

Ingredients:

1 head of cauliflower
2-3 Tbsp of Ghee/butter
1-1 ½ cups of heavy cream or unsweetened almond milk
1 tsp salt
1 tsp pepper
1 tsp granulated garlic

Roasting the cauliflower in the oven first and then combining ingredients adds incredible flavor, but it certainly takes longer to prepare.

For the sake of getting in and out of the kitchen in 2 hours, start by putting the cleaned cauliflower in a microwave safe dish, adding a small amount of water to the bottom of the dish. Cover with plastic wrap and cook on high 3-4 minutes, repeating this process until the cauliflower is easily punctured with a fork. Remove and allow to cool for a few minutes (still want it to be warm). Then break up into smaller pieces.

In a food processor or Ninja©, place the cauliflower, add 1/2 of the milk, butter, and season with salt, pepper, and granulated garlic; pulse until it becomes smooth. Continue to add milk until the mixture resembles a mashed potato-like consistency. Can add additional ghee or butter to serve, and additional seasonings to taste.

Chicken Pho

Typically, it takes hours to obtain that perfect blend of spices and yummy pho broth goodness, but when you find something that makes prepping easy, well, you go with it! This takes no time at all to get this together, and if you stack the ingredients into a mason jar and the broth in another jar, it is a great lunch on the go!

Ingredients:

3 organic cooked chicken breasts from slow cooker (cooked for Shawarma)
1 container of Pho Broth
1 pkg. Angel Hair made from Konjac tuber
2 carrots (preferably purple and yellow)
1/2 jalapeno
6-8 springs of cilantro
2 Tbsp organic bacon bits
1/2 yellow onion
Mung sprouts (optional)
1 wedge lime
Tamari or soy sauce

Heat pho broth thoroughly on med/low heat, then simmer. While pho is heating, make noodles with carrots, slice jalapeno thinly and put aside. Cut chicken breast against grain into 1/4 inch slices. Prepare the angel hair noodles per the instructions on the packaging.

In a deep soup bowl (they make really cool pho bowls!) put the angel noodles, carrot noodles, warm chicken breast, and all other ingredients into the pho bowl. Pour the hot pho broth onto the ingredients; season with tamari or siracha, curl up and enjoy!

Roasted Broccoli

Broccoli is a great side dish for any main course. It has lots of fiber, with very little carbohydrates and as a dark green vegetable, it provides lots of great vitamins. Super easy to cook, you simply cut it up, season it to your liking, put it in the oven, and let it go! Really a yummy side that works with anything.

Ingredients:

2 large broccoli heads or 1 large bag of broccoli florets (hint: go with the bag!)
2 tsp of salt
1 tsp ground ginger
1 tsp black pepper
1/2 tsp red pepper flakes
3 Tbsp ghee or organic butter
1 Tbsp sesame oil

Preheat the oven to 400 degrees F.

Place the broccoli florets in a mixing bowl and pour the oil and melted butter over them. Mix thoroughly to ensure that all florets are coated in the oil/butter mixture. Pour the florets into the disposable aluminum pan and then generously sprinkle with the seasonings, salt, pepper and pepper flakes. Place in oven and cook for 45 minutes to 1 hour or until the cauliflower has browned slightly and is soft when punctured with fork. This can be topped with a shredded hard cheese or can be accompanied with a feta whipped yogurt cream or just by itself!

Miso Seared Tuna Bowl

Ingredients:

2 tuna steaks (approx. 1 lb)
Apple cider and ginger sesame dressing
Small bag of matchstick carrots
1 cup of sliced almonds
1 bag of frozen cauliflower fried rice
1 avocado
Siracha pepper
1 bunch cilantro (optional)
Black and white sesame seed sprinkles

2 Dry organic miso packets
1 cucumber
1 bag of Asian slaw salad
1 lime
1 bunch green onions
Salt/pepper for seasoning
Granulated garlic
1 jalapeno pepper (opt.)
2 Tbsp roasted sesame oil

Place fresh, cleaned tuna in Ziplock or sealed container and add approximately 1 cup of marinade to tuna; place in fridge for approximately 30-45 minutes.

While tuna is marinating, peel cucumber, then cut in small cubes; add 1-2 cups of matchstick carrots to cucumbers into mixing bowl and blend together, then set aside. Cut avocado in half, remove seed and slice thinly in skin; then remove with spoon (see essentials video if needed). Cut the lime in half, then slice. Squeeze section of lime over avocado slices to avoid browning.

Arrange clean Asian chopped slaw into a large individual serving bowl into one area. Do the same with the cucumber, carrot mixture and place next to the slaw. Lay the avocado over the slaw. Place the bowl in the fridge and remove the tuna. Next, heat the frozen fried rice in microwave according to the directions. Once completed, remove from microwave and set aside to cool slightly. On a hot griddle, pour 1 Tbsp of sesame oil onto griddle or large flat frying pan and place the tuna onto surface; do not move. Cook approximately 4-5 minutes per side and remove. You want the tuna to be seared and pink inside. Cut in strips, place over the veggies, and garnish with cilantro, green onions and sesame seeds. Let the drooling begin!

Easy Pizza Frittata

Ingredients:

8 large organic eggs
1 sweet yellow onion
1 pkg of organic/no antibiotic pepperoni slices
1 Tbsp minced garlic
1 small bag of baby spinach
1/2 tsp fresh ground nutmeg (you will thank me later!)
1/2 handful of sliced porcini mushrooms
2 tsp dried oregano or Italian seasoning
2 Tbsp unsweetened almond milk or organic milk
Salt/pepper to taste
1/2 cup of shredded mozzarella or buffalo mozzarella (small round balls)
Grated parmesan (optional)
1 Tbsp olive oil

Dice the onion and set aside; ensure spinach is washed and dried thoroughly before use. In an oven proof skillet, (This part is very important, DO NOT put a skillet in the oven if it is not noted oven proof. You can use a ceramic pie pan for this recipe if skillet is unavailable.) Pour olive oil in pan and then add onions. Cook, stirring occasionally until onions are translucent, approximately 5 minutes; add mushrooms and cook until mushrooms have lost most of the moisture, then add the spinach. Cook until the spinach is wilted, approximately 2-3 minutes. Season with salt and pepper.

In a large bowl, whisk together eggs, Italian seasoning, milk, and season with salt and pepper; then finely grate nutmeg into the mixture. Pour the mixture over vegetables and cook until the edge of the eggs separate from pan, approximately 4-5 minutes. Add the pepperoni and cheese, then transfer the skillet to the oven and cook for approximately 5-7 minutes. Remove from oven, sprinkle parmesan onto frittata and let sit for an additional 5 minutes. Cut in wedges and serve with mixed greens or roasted veggies!!

Sweet Potato Fries

This is a great substitution for traditional fries; now do they have carbs, well of course! However, they are high in fiber and full of vitamins and nutrients, so eating (your portion size) every now and then can still produce great results, while feeding the need for a fry or two!

Ingredients:

2 large sweet potatoes
1 Tbsp olive oil or coconut oil, melted
1 tsp sea salt
1 tsp pepper
1 tsp smoked paprika
1/2 tsp chili powder
1/2 tsp onion powder
1 tsp granulated garlic
1/4 tsp ground cinnamon
1/2 cup grated parmesan
1 Tbsp dried oregano

Preheat oven to 400 degrees. In a small mixing bowl, combine all dry ingredients together and set aside. Cut the cleaned sweet potato into fries that are approximately 3 inches x 1/2 inch (a mandolin can be used here, but the fries can still be cut manually).

Place fries into a large mixing bowl and coat well with oil. Sprinkle 1/2 of the dry mixture onto the fries and mix well with hands (yes, this is messy!) until all is well coated; then place in a single layer on parchment lined baking sheet. Sprinkle the remaining dry seasonings onto the fries and place in oven. Bake for approximately 35-40 minutes, turning the baking sheet half way through the cooking process. When the fries are crispy but soft when punctured with fork, they are ready to go! Remove from oven and sprinkle with dried oregano and parmesan to garnish.

This goes great with burgers, wings, and even frittata!

PLAY BY PLAY
WEEK FOUR
6 Week PREP FOR IT START UP COURSE

Is prepping for the week starting to feel like second nature? Maybe getting into a bit of a rhythm? By week four, you should be feeling more comfortable in the kitchen and have begun to strategically set up the pantry for easy grab and go, making the prepping process far more streamlined. Keep it up! Again, prior to starting the prep process for week four, make sure you have worked through the PEER steps (Prep, Eat, Evaluate, Repeat) to provide you with the greatest chance for success.

Bullet Points:
- The meals that take longer to prepare and cook should be started on first.
- Review the weekly menu and collect all of the ingredients, condiments, and seasonings. Sort with each individual dish/tray.
- Wash all vegetables first to expedite the prep.
- Clean utensils and kitchen equipment as you go to minimize the cleaning in the end.

Supplies:
Parchment Paper	Aluminum Pans (3-4)	Slow cooker
Skillet x 2	Cookie Sheets	Mixing bowls (med, large)
Prep/storage container	Spatula	Tongs x 2
Cutting knives	Cutting board (plastic/wood)	Measuring cups/spoons
Ziplock bags	Whisk or fork	Timer

- Preheat oven 400 degrees
- Sort all the ingredients with the specific recipes, trays or pans.
- Place chicken breast, in slow cooker add onions, and water cook on high.
- Chop the onions, bacon, beets, broccoli, mushrooms, etc. Separate into different dishes and put aside.
- In a heated skillet put in olive oil and cook bacon, onions, and mushrooms until browned and put in a bowl allowing to cool.
- In a Ziplock bag put cleaned tuna steaks and add the marinade from recipe, seal and put in the fridge.
- In a large mixing bowl put broccoli, olive oil and seasoning, mixing together with tongs and place on 1 half of a parchment lined cookie sheet.

WHAT'S EATING YOU?

- In the same mixing bowl put the okra or green beans in bowl, adding olive oil and seasonings and mix with tongs. Then layer on the other half of the parchment lined cookie sheet and place in oven.
- Assemble all of the miso tuna ingredients and veggies in the storage or prep container and set aside. Take the tuna streaks out of the fridge, pat dry and season per recipe. In a heated skillet sear the tuna according to the recipe and once seared on both sides remove and set on a plate to rest for a few minutes. Slice the tuna into ¼ inch slices and place over the vegetable bowl storage or prep container.
- Take the cooled bacon, onion and mushroom mixture and combine with the ground meat adding ingredients according to the recipe. Put into bread/loaf aluminum pan. Put sauce and bacon strips on top and but in the oven.
- In a medium mixing bowl put the cubed beets, olive oil and seasonings according to recipe and place on a small parchment lined cookie sheet or aluminum pan and put in oven.
- In a heated skillet put olive oil and cook the cauliflower rice with pine nuts and turmeric following the recipe, when done transfer to prep or storage container and allow to cool.
- Remove the chicken breast from the slow cooker, drain on a paper towel lined plate and when cool slice into ¼ inch slices. Half of the chicken will be put into mason jars for pho and other half will be used to cook chicken shawarma.
- In a mason jar, place the chicken and follow recipe adding the remaining pho ingredients excluding the broth, secure the lid and place in the fridge. Pour broth into another mason jar and place in the fridge.
- In a heated, oiled skillet add the other ½ of chicken and ingredients following the shawarma recipe when completely cooked allow to cool and place over the turmeric rice in the prep or storage container and place in the fridge.
- Remove the broccoli and okra or green beans from oven, allow to cool and then place in prep or storage containers. Check the meatloaf and if ready remove and let cool.
- In a nonstick skillet, sauté the frittata ingredients, mix the egg mixture gently and set aside. Pour the egg mixture over the skillet vegetable and follow the recipe.
- Put the cleaned cauliflower head into the microwave according to the recipe and steam until soft. Follow the recipe and complete the mashed cauliflower per recipe and place in prep or storage container. Pick up all disposable equipment, utensils and wash remaining dishes and bowls.

WEEK FIVE

BOLOGNESE MEAT SAUCE
WITH ROASTED SPAGHETTI SQUASH OR PALM NOODLES

PISTACHIO AND PORK RIND PANKO CRUSTED SALMON
WITH AVOCADO SALAD

BARBACOA BEEF WITH FIX INS
AND SWEET POTATO MASH

MONGOLIAN CHICKEN
WITH CAULIFLOWER RICE AND ROASTED GREEN BEANS

SWEDISH MEATBALLS
WITH ROASTED BUTTERNUT SQUASH

WHAT'S EATING YOU?

6 Week PREP FOR IT START UP COURSE
WEEK 5

Congratulations! Making your way into week 5, you have started to perfect those essential prepping skills. We will turn up the heat (just a little!) and try a few slightly more complex recipes. But, Oh! How they will taste! The goal is still to get in and out of the kitchen within 2 hours. Before heading to the grocery check the essentials list to ensure you are stocked and ready for the week! Again, remember organic when available.

Meat:
1 pound organic ground beef
1 pound organic ground pork or mild Italian sausage
2- salmon filets (approx 4-6 oz)
2 pounds of organic beef tips
1 pack (4) boneless, skinless chicken thighs
1 bag organic Italian turkey meatballs

Fresh Vegetables:
1 spaghetti squash or 1 can palm linguini noodles
2-sweet potatoes
1 cauliflower head
1 avocados
1 butternut squash whole or cubed
1 lb fresh/frozen green beans
2 yellow onions (bag from last week)
4 carrots
2 jalapeno
2 lime
2 bunch cilantro
½ pound porcini or cremini mushrooms
1 navel orange
1 package of red cabbage slaw (with carrots)
1 red pepper

Condiments, Seasoning, Oils:
Mexican cheese for barbacoa beef (optional)
2 dried ancho chilis
blocked or shredded Parmesan Cheese
2 large cans San Marzano whole tomatoes
Unsweetened almond milk or organic milk
1 container almond milk sour cream or organic
1 contain Konjac® noodles
½ cup roasted chopped peanuts or slivered almonds
1 small container of organic peanut or almond butter
1 small container Cajun seasoning (this can be made)
1 bunch scallions
1 small section fresh ginger

Breakfast foods: Repeat week 2

Spaghetti Sauce with Spaghetti Squash Noodles

Ingredients:

3 Tbsp olive oil (1 Tbsp for squash) 1 medium sweet yellow onion
2-3 medium organic carrots 1 tsp pepper
1 tsp salt 1 Tbsp minced garlic
2 Tbsp roasted tomato paste 1/4-1/2 cup of dry sherry
2 cans organic peeled tomatoes 2 Tbsp dried Italian seasoning
1 bay leaf 1 med/large spaghetti squash
1 Tbsp oregano or 3 fresh sprigs of oregano
Grated organic parmesan cheese or vegan substitute
5 fresh basil leaves, chiffon or diced

Preheat the oven to 400 degrees F.

Clean and dry 1 spaghetti squash; poke holes in the squash with a fork and place in the microwave for about 1 minute. Cut the squash in half lengthwise and scrape out the seeds and inside of the squash. Brush with olive oil; salt and pepper the inside portion of the squash and place on a parchment lined baking sheet with opening facing down. Roast in the oven for approximately 30 minutes or when fork punctures skin easily.

Heat 1 Tbsp of olive oil in a large sauce pan or 2-quart pot on medium heat and add onions and carrots; add salt and pepper, sweating them until the onions become slightly translucent, about 8-10 minutes, stirring occasionally. Add garlic and brown for 2-3 more minutes; then add tomato paste, stirring for approximately 10 more minutes. Add sherry and deglaze the pan. Add tomatoes, dried basil, Italian seasoning, and bay leaf. Cover and cook on low heat for about 25-30 minutes, adding water or chicken broth as needed. You can add additional salt and pepper to taste.

While tomato sauce is cooking, brown 1 pound of ground turkey or ground organic beef; salt and pepper to taste, then drain. Using an emulsifier or blender, emulsify the tomato sauce until thick sauce is noted; then add the cooked meat to the sauce and cook for an additional 10 minutes. Add milk and half of cheese to the sauce and stir to avoid sticking to bottom of pot. Take cooled squash and using a fork, loosen the inside of the squash, making noodles and keep them in the squash skin. Scoop approx. 1 cup of sauce and pour into the squash, mixing with the squash noodles. Top with parmesan cheese or substitute and place back into the oven for 5 min, sprinkle basil over the squash and enjoy!

Pistachio Crusted Salmon

Ingredients:

2 large filets of salmon (4 x 6-inch slab, wild caught preferred)
1 large navel orange, zested and juiced
1 cup of Pork rind Panko Crumbs
1 cup of minced pistachios
1 tsp fresh or dried thyme
1 tsp fresh or dried minced oregano
3 Tbsp of almond flour (1 Tbsp to be used in the pecan mixture)
1 organic egg, lightly beaten
1-2 tsp of salt
1/2 to 1 tsp of cayenne pepper
1 tsp granulated garlic
3 Tbsp ghee (clarified butter 1 ½ to use for cooking and 1 ½ to drizzle on cooked fish)
1 Tbsp fresh parsley

Place the almond flour in a shallow dish and season with salt, pepper, and granulated garlic, then thoroughly mix flour with a fork. In a shallow bowl, slightly whisk 1 egg with orange juice and sprinkle with salt and pepper. In 3rd shallow dish, mix remaining almond flour, minced pistachios, orange zest, thyme and oregano, thoroughly seasoning again with salt pepper and granulated garlic. Dredge, (pull the filet through the flour and then flip over and coat the opposite site) shaking off any excess. Then dredge the filet through the egg mixture, ensuring that it is coated well. Allow the excess to fall back into the egg mixture. Then dredge this filet into the pecan mixture and push the ingredients down onto the filet, making sure it covers all parts of the fish. Place on a clean plate and heat your frying pan or griddle to medium heat. Add 1 ½ of the ghee to the pan and allow it to melt and coat the entire pan. You can substitute olive oil here, but it will not be as decadent! When the ghee is melted, (do not let this brown too much, or it will burn and can cause the fish to taste burnt) Place the filets into the pan and press down with a spatula. DO NOT move the filets, allowing them to cook on the first side for at least 3-5 minutes. Carefully release the filet from the pan with the spatula and flip over to the uncooked side and cook for an additional 3-5 minutes. Salmon will be slightly darker pink in the middle. Remove filets and place on a clean plate. Wipe the pan with a clean paper towel and then add the remaining ghee with the fresh parsley and stir for about 2-3 minutes. Drizzle this mixture over the filets prior to serving. Super easy prep with tons of flavor.

Avocado Salad

Super easy salad to put together with plenty of good fats, flavor, and is a great complement to our hearty fish dish!

Ingredients:

2 avocados
1 cup of heirloom cherry tomatoes, cut in half
1/2 Purple/red onion, chopped
Fresh bunch of parsley
Fresh bunch of thyme
1 tsp minced garlic
1 tsp salt
1 tsp pepper

Dressing:
1 Tbsp apple cider vinegar
1 Tbsp sesame oil
1/2 tsp salt
1 Tbsp honey
1 tsp grated fresh ginger

Whisk the dressing ingredients together in a large measuring cup and put aside.

Cut the avocado in half, core and cut into cubes (following the recommendations from the Essentials 101 video for an easy way to cut an avocado). Cut the cherry tomatoes in half and chop the onion. Mince the parsley and pull leaves off of the thyme stems, then mix all of the ingredients in a large mixing bowl. Once combined, pour the dressing over the vegetables, mixing well. This can be served immediately, but taste improves when allowed to rest in the fridge for at least an hour.

Barbacoa Beef

This is such an amazing dish! What makes this dish so flavorful is the marinade that you combine before putting it into the slow cooker or oven. Even though it seems like several ingredients, you just throw them all into the food processor and blend them up; takes very little time, and yields an amazing flavor!

Ingredients:

3-4 dried ancho chili peppers
1/4 cup olive or avocado oil
4-5 whole garlic cloves peeled or 2 Tbsp minced garlic
2 tsp salt/pepper
1 lime, juiced
1 onion (1/2 for sauce)
1 Tbsp dried oregano or 1 small punch of fresh oregano
2 tsp cumin
5-7 cloves or 1 tsp ground cloves
2 cups beef broth
1-2 cups water
1 bunch cilantro
1 cup dry cooking sherry, preferably organic
Organic beef stew chunks or beef roast (approx. 2 lbs.)
Braising seasoning (1tsp each of granulated garlic, onion powder, smoked paprika, ground cumin, ground coffee)
1 Tbsp sifted almond flour

In food processor or ninja, combine first 11 ingredients until a thick sauce is noted. Put sauce aside. Dry the beef stew chunks or roast and coat with braising seasoning on all sides. Brown the meat in medium pot on medium heat until golden brown; remove from pot. Using 1 cup of sherry, deglaze the pot and then add 1 cup of beef broth cook for approximately 5 minutes; remove from the heat. Place prepared meat into the slow cooker, add remainder of onion over meat, and pour the liquid from the pot onto the meat; add the sauce ancho mixture to the slow cooker. Cook on high for 1-2 hours and then on low heat for approximately 4-5 hours until meat falls apart or pulls apart with fork.

Savory Sweet Potato Mash

Such a hearty, savory side dish with plenty of fiber and flavor to boot! If you are striving to continue eating healthy during the holidays, this is a great substitution for the traditional sweet potato dish.

Ingredients:

2 sweet potatoes, cleaned and baked
1/2 cup of unflavored almond milk or organic cream cheese
1 Tbsp Honey
2 Tbsp ghee or organic butter, melted
1/4 tsp organic vanilla
1 Tbsp minced garlic
1 bunch green onions
1 Tbsp of fresh minced/finely chopped parsley
1/2 tsp salt
1/2 tsp pepper

Remove the potato skins from the baked sweet potatoes and discard. Place the sweet potato flesh into a mixing bowl and mash with a potato masher or hand-mixer on lowest setting. Add the green onions and parsley; continue to blend and then add cream cheese, honey, butter, vanilla and salt and pepper to taste.

Mongolian Chicken

Such an easy dish to assemble and turns out perfect every time. Great with cauliflower rice or even combination fried cauliflower rice.

Ingredients:

4-6 boneless, skinless chicken thighs
Tapioca (potato) starch approx. 2 Tbsp
1 cup of coconut sugar or 1/2 cup of monk sweetener
1 cup of tamari sauce (organic soy sauce)
1 cup water
3 dried chili peppers
2 tsp salt
2 tsp pepper
2 Tbsp minced garlic
1/4 cup of coconut aminos
1/2 bag of matchstick carrots (left over from last week)
1 cup of diced scallions

If cooking in the conventional oven, preheat oven to 400 F. Can be cooked in oven or slow cooker. Clean and dry chicken, cutting into 1–2-inch strips and place in bowl. Sprinkle with tapioca starch, salt and pepper; stir to completely cover all chicken. Place in a 9x13 aluminum pan or in slow cooker. Sprinkle carrots over chicken. In a separate mixing bowl, combine coconut sugar, tamari, water, coconut aminos, and dried chili peppers. Pour over chicken and cook on low for 3-4 hours in slow cooker or approximately 1 ½ hours in the oven, covered with aluminum foil. Remove aluminum foil 30-40 minutes before cooking is done. Serve over cauliflower rice.

Roasted Asian Green Beans

Everyone, well, almost everyone loves green beans, but finding new ways to serve these great green vegetables can be challenging. Roasting green beans is a great way to bring out the unique flavors in the beans, and adding a few simple ingredients draws the additional flavors out even more!

Ingredients:

1 lb of fresh green beans, cut and cleaned
1 Tbsp roasted sesame oil
1-2 tsp tamari or organic soy sauce
1 tsp Chinese chili paste
1 Tbsp almond butter or peanut butter
1 Tbsp Rice Wine Vinegar
1 tsp roasted sesame seeds

Preheat the oven to 400 degrees F.

In a large measuring cup, add all of the seasonings and wet ingredients, and whisk until butter is completely dissolved. In a mixing bowl, place the cleaned green beans and pour the wet ingredients over the beans, mixing well. Using tongs, place onto parchment lined baking sheet. Place in oven and roast for approximately 30-35 minutes until the beans are soft, but not mushy. Remove and garnish with sesame seeds if desired.

Swedish Meatballs over Zoodles

Ingredients:

1 bag organic chicken or turkey meatballs (frozen)
1 Tbsp Olive oil
1 small onion, diced
1 Tbsp ghee
1 Tbsp sifted almond or coconut flour
1/2 tsp allspice
1/2 tsp honey (preferred) or monk fruit sweetener
1/2 tsp nutmeg (grated from whole nutmeg you should still have)
1 tsp grey Poupon or organic brown mustard
1 cup of almond milk sour cream
1 cup of beef broth
1 Tbsp organic dry cooking sherry
Fresh parsley for garnish

I suggest slightly thawing meatballs and make sure they are dry prior to browning. In a heated skillet, put 1 Tbsp olive oil and brown the meatballs well on all sides. Remove and drain on a paper towel covered plate. Melt 1Ttbsp of ghee or butter in the pan; add the fine almond flour or coconut flour and stir constantly for approximately 3 minutes; then add onion and continue to cook until translucent, stirring occasionally. Deglaze pan with the sherry, then add the beef broth, stirring until smooth; add sour cream or cream cheese. Season with spices, honey, nutmeg salt, pepper and grey Poupon mustard. Return the meatballs back into the mixture and allow to simmer on low for approximately 15 minutes. Meanwhile, cook the noodles in the microwave or on the stove top until soft; then pour the meatball sauce over the zoodles and garnish with the fresh parsley.

Roasted Butternut Squash

Butternut has become a staple vegetable in our home since this wellness and weight loss journey began. It is such a high fiber, versatile, and very flavorful veggie. When roasted, it allows the flavor to caramelize on the outside with a soft buttery inside. Very hearty and comforting dish!

Ingredients:

1 large butternut squash, peeled and cubed, or already cubed squash
1 Tbsp roasted olive oil
1 tsp salt
1 tsp granulated garlic
1 tsp onion powder
1/2 tsp chili pepper
1/2 tsp ground cinnamon
1 tsp smoked paprika
1 Tbsp dried parsley
1 tsp dried rosemary
2 Tbsp grated parmesan and 1 Tbsp fresh parsley for garnish (optional)

Preheat the oven to 400 degrees F.

In a mixing bowl, place the cleaned, cubed butternut squash, pour olive oil over the vegetables and mix well with tongs. In a separate smaller mixing bowl, mix all dry ingredients together and sprinkle over the butternut squash; mix well with tongs and then place single layer onto parchment lined baking sheet. Place in oven and roast for approximately 40-50 minutes until squash is browned and fork is able to puncture squash easily. Remove and this can be garnished with fresh parsley and rosemary and even some grated parmesan.

WHAT'S EATING YOU?

PLAY BY PLAY
WEEK FIVE

6 Week PREP FOR IT START UP COURSE

By week five you are likely getting really great sea-legs and may not even need the play-by-play instructions. However, just as a coach provides resources along the way, the play-by-play will help to facilitate your success. Remember to worked through the PEER steps (Prep, Eat, Evaluate, Repeat) to provide you with the greatest chance for success.

Bullet Points:

- The meals that take longer to prepare and cook should be started on first.
- Review the weekly menu and collect all of the ingredients, condiments, and seasonings. Sort with each individual dish/tray.
- Wash all vegetables first to expedite the prep.
- Clean utensils and kitchen equipment as you go to minimize the cleaning in the end.

Supplies:

Parchment Paper	Aluminum Pans (3-4)	Slow cooker
Skillet x 2	Cookie Sheets	Mixing bowls (med, large)
Prep/storage container	Spatula	Tongs x 2
Cutting knives	Cutting board (plastic/wood)	Measuring cups/spoons
Ziplock bags	Whisk or fork	Timer
Vegetable scraper	Dutch oven	Emulsifier or blender
Grater	Ice cream scoop	Boiling pot

- Preheat oven 400 degrees. Sort all the ingredients with the specific recipes, trays or pans.

- Take beef chunks and season according to the recipe put aside. In a blender, mix the ingredients for the sauce until well blended and put aside.

- Cut onion slices, chopped onions, carrots, cube butternut, jalapeno, etc. Set aside in separate dishes.

- Take cleaned sweet potatoes, poking with fork or paring knife, wrap in foil and put on a parchment lined cookie sheet then place in oven.

- Heat olive oil in a Dutch oven and braise beef chunks. Follow recipe to deglaze the pot. Place the beef chunks into the slow cooker and then add the sliced onions, beef gravy. Cover and turn on high for approximately 1 hour.

- Clean chicken and cut into think strips and put in a zip lock bag. Add the starch, seal and place in the fridge.

- Put the butternut squash into mixing bowl and add olive oil, spices and seasonings. Mix with tongs and then place on parchment lined cookie sheet and put in the oven.
- Make the Asian noodle salad according to recipe. Take the chicken and empty into an aluminum pan and add ingredients and mix with tongs in pan. Cover and put in the oven.
- In a Dutch oven, heat olive oil, chopped onion and carrots and follow the Bolognese recipe. When put on simmer, move to the next task.
- Cut spaghetti squash in half and core out the seeds and remove seeds. Brush the halves with olive oil, salt and pepper. Place them face down on parchment lined aluminum pan and set aside. After Bolognese has cooked turn off to let it cool.
- Put salted water in boiling pot and bring to a boil. Place the washed, halved Brussel sprouts in boiling water. Par-boil for approx. 5 minutes transfer to strainer and allow to dry. Then in a mixing bowl put the Brussel sprouts, olive oil and seasonings. Mix well with tongs and add to a parchment lined cookie sheet. Add bacon cubes to the BS and then put in oven. Check chicken, uncover and cook for approximately 10 more minutes.
- In skillet brown turkey meatballs put on napkin-lined plate to drain. In the same skillet add more olive oil and remaining ingredients for Swedish meatballs and when all ingredients combined, add meatballs into the sauce cook according to the recipe.
- Put spaghetti squash in the oven. Emulsify or blend the cooled spaghetti sauce until a thick sauce noted. (Take the bay leaf out first) Add milk and cheese to the sauce and simmer for approximately 10 minutes and then allow to cool.
- Season salmon and sear in skillet on both sides when done put on plate and allow to cool, place in prep container with Asian noodle.
- Remove the butternut squash, when able to insert a fork easily and allow to cool. Once cool place in prep or storage container. Add Swedish meatballs to the butternut squash in the prep or storage container and put in the fridge.
- Remove sweet potatoes allow to cool and store in containers. Remove spaghetti squash allow to cool and shred into the prep container then add sauce. (Put some sauce in a Ziplock back and put in freezer for next week prep)
- Check on Brussel sprouts, put shredded parmesan or asiago cheese to Brussel sprouts and allow to cook for an additional 10 minutes then remove. Allow to cool and store in prep or storage container. ·Pick up all disposable equipment, utensils and wash remaining dishes and bowls.

WEEK SIX

STUFFED PEPPERS
WITH ROASTED BRUSSEL SPROUTS AND BACON

CHICKEN CACCIATORE
WITH SPAGHETTI SQUASH OR PALM NOODLES AND ROASTED KALE

CHICKEN AND SAUSAGE JAMBALAYA
WITH OKRA FRIES

SHEPARD'S PIE
WITH ROASTED BROCCOLI

CAULIFLOWER PIZZA
WITH MUFFULETTA BROCCOLI SALAD

WHAT'S EATING YOU?

6 Week PREP FOR IT START UP COURSE
WEEK 6

YOU are finally here! You made it to the last week of the 6-week PREP FOR IT start-up course! It takes time and massive effort to create this kind of discipline in your life, and you will reap the dividends from this hard work! You are doing a new you and we are thrilled to be able to equip you will the tools and the encouragement you need to reach your goal of wellness and weight loss! Now let's get that last grocery list and go for it! Remember to check on your condiments, cans and oil inventory to cut cost!

Meat:
1 ½ pounds of organic ground beef
1 pd organic pork
½ pd ground mild Italian or chorizo sausage
3 organic chicken legs and thighs (bone and skin)
1 Rotisserie Chicken (1/2 for recipe/half for off night)
1 small pk. organic andouille chicken sausage
1 small pack organic pepperoni slices

Fresh Vegetables:
1 spaghetti squash or 1 can palm linguini noodles
3 carrots
1 lb or bag of Brussel sprouts
3 head cauliflower or 1 head and 2 bags, riced
4 yellow onions
1 bundle of asparagus
1 container organic spring mix
½ pound of cremini or porcini mushrooms
1 yellow squash and 1 zucchini
1 bag of broccoli florets
2 bell peppers (yellow or red)
1 small eggplant (thin Japanese)

Condiments, Seasoning, Oils:
1 can tomato paste
1 carton chicken broth
1 block gruyere or white cheddar cheese
2 can organic tomatoes diced/chopped
Dried/fresh parsley
1 can harissa (optional)
Ground cardamom
Small asiago cheese wedge
1 small container of organic mozzarella cheese
1 small package of fresh basil
1 frozen cauliflower pizza crust
1 small container of marinated black olives

Breakfast foods: Repeat week 3

Chorizo, Eggplant and Cauliflower Rice Stuffed Bell Peppers

We have taken our traditional Southern Stuffed Peppers and added a Moroccan twist to this great staple. It's hearty, spicy and savory, making this a wonderful main dish.

Ingredients:

2 medium to large yellow or orange peppers

1/2 lb of ground chorizo (seasoned pork)

1 small yellow onion, diced

2 tsp granulated garlic

2 Tbsp tomato paste or tomato relish (harissa)

1/3 cup of cooking sherry or water

1/4 tsp cinnamon

1/2 tsp cayenne pepper (omit if using chorizo)

1/3 cup of chicken broth

1 head cauliflower, minced or finely diced (can substitute bag of cauliflower rice here)

1/2 lb of organic ground beef

small Japanese eggplant, diced

1 Tbsp minced garlic

2 tsp onion powder

1 Tbsp olive oil

1/4 tsp cardamom

1 tsp pepper

1 tsp salt

Asiago or parmesan cheese organic approx. 1 cup (optional for keto and modified clean eating plan)

Preheat oven to 400 F. Cut tops off peppers and remove the seeds and rind inside of the peppers; set aside. In large skillet, heat olive oil and sauté onions, minced garlic, eggplant, salt and pepper for 5 minutes or until onions are sweating. Stir in granulated garlic, onion powder, and tomato relish; cook for another 5 minutes; add sherry and deglaze pan. Add organic ground beef and chorizo into mixture and brown. No need to drain if using low fat ground meat, but if using regular ground meat, brown in separate pan, drain and then add to skillet.

Add half of minced cauliflower and stir into the mixture, then add additional cauliflower. Can add 1/2 cup of cheese into the mixture and then stuff all peppers. Add additional cheese to the tops of peppers, place peppers into baking pans with small amount of water to cover just the bottom of the pan. Bake for approximately 30 minutes or until peppers are soft and can be pierced with fork easily.

Roasted Brussel Sprouts with Bacon

Literally one of my all-time favorite dishes! Obviously, bacon makes everything better, but the bacon in this dish brings the Brussel sprouts to a whole other level! The key to this dish is the par-boiling (precooking the Brussel sprouts in boiling water before roasting). This allows them to soften up enough to get caramelized in the oven when roasting.

Ingredients:

1 lb of Brussel sprouts, halved and cleaned (I usually cut the stem off.)
1/2 lb of bacon
1 Tbsp granulated garlic
1-2 Tbsp olive oil
1-2 tsp salt
1-2 tsp pepper
Shaved or shredded parmesan (optional before serving)

Preheat the oven on roast at 400 degrees F. Boil water in medium pot and salt the water generously. In batches, if necessary, boil the halved Brussel sprouts for approximately 8-10 minutes. (They should still be very green, but becoming soft). Remove and strain off water, then transfer into a disposable aluminum pan. Drizzle with olive oil and mix thoroughly. Add salt, pepper, and granulated garlic, and stir again. Cut the bacon into small 1/4 inch cubes (easier done if the bacon is cut immediately after removing from the fridge) and spread over the top of the Brussel sprouts. Place in oven uncovered and roast for approximately 45 minutes, stirring occasionally. The sprouts are done when the edges are browning and the bacon appears brown and done. Remove from the oven; can garnish with shredded parmesan over the Brussel sprouts.

Not Ya' Mama's Chicken Cacciatore

Ingredients:

2 each organic chicken thighs and legs (bone in)	1 dry bay leaf
1 Tbsp sifted almond flour	1 tsp sweet paprika
1-2 Tbsp olive oil	1-2 tsp coarse sea salt
1 onion, thinly sliced	1-2 tsp pepper to taste
1 zucchini and 1 squash, cubed	1 tsp cayenne pepper
Porcini mushrooms, approx. 10	1 Tbsp minced garlic
2 Tbsp roasted organic tomato paste	1 tsp granulated garlic

1 large can Sans Marzano Roma tomatoes, drained
1/2 cup of organic red wine or sherry
1 cup of organic chicken broth
1-2 Tbsp dried Italian seasoning
1/3 cup of marinated black olives, pitted
3-4 basil leaves, chiffon

Preheat the oven to 400 degrees F. Clean and dry, salt and pepper chicken, and dust with flour. Heat 1 Tbsp of oil in a large Dutch pot and brown chicken approximately 5-7 minutes on each side. Remove from oil. Add additional oil to heated pot; add onions, carrots and cook for approximately 5-8 minutes until translucent and slightly brown; season with salt and pepper. Add garlic, bay leaf and cook for approximately 1-3 minutes longer. Add mushrooms and stir additional 3-5 minutes, seasoning as needed. Add tomato paste and cook on medium heat while stirring; add additional seasonings and continue to cook on medium, stirring until the mixture becomes a dark brown/red color. (Make sure to constantly stir the mixture to avoid sticking) Add sherry and deglaze the pan with wooden spoon, slowly adding the beef broth a little at a time to create a thick sauce. Add zucchini and squash, cayenne and granulated garlic at this time. Cover and reduce to low heat, adding chicken broth as needed to maintain a thick consistency, but to avoid burning or drying out the mixture. Add tomatoes and add to the sauce, breaking apart into large chunks with wooden spatula. When mixture comes to a boil, place browned chicken back into the pot and simmer for an additional 20-30 minutes or until the chicken pulls away from bone. Add olives and cook an additional 5-7 minutes; add fresh basil and oregano and serve over spaghetti squash.

Roasted Kale

This is a very easy recipe and tastes similar to the kale chips, but is not as crispy so it complements very hearty meals, allowing you to get your greens in a flavorful way!

Ingredients:

1 large bag of kale pieces (washed and dried)
1 tsp of olive oil
1 tsp of granulated garlic
1 tsp salt
1 tsp pepper
1 Tbsp grated parmesan

Preheat the oven on roast at 400 degrees.

Remove any tough stems from kale pieces and place the completely dried kale into a mixing bowl; coat with the olive oil and then massage the leaves to coat all leaves well. Spread the leaves out onto the parchment lined baking sheet and then sprinkle the seasonings over all of the leaves. Place in the oven and bake for approximately 20-25 minutes, checking them often to ensure they are not overcooked or burnt. Remove and can be eaten with grated parmesan or asiago cheese.

Chicken and Sausage Jambalaya

This is a wonderful alternative to the high carbohydrate and starchy Cajun staple. All of the great flavors with just a fraction of the calories! Great meal!

Ingredients:

1 full head cauliflower (pulsed to rice size) or right rice (preferred)
1 small pack or 2 links of andouille sausage or pork sausage
1/2 diced leftover rotisserie chicken
2 celery stalks, diced
1 yellow or orange pepper, diced
2 Tbsp minced garlic
1 tsp pepper (to taste)
1 Tbsp dried or fresh oregano
2 Tbsp minced fresh parsley
1-2 cups of chicken broth
1 can of diced roasted tomatoes
1 tsp cayenne pepper (omit if using andouille)
1 onion, minced
2-3 tsp salt (to taste)
1 Tbsp dried/fresh thyme
1-2 tsp granulated garlic
1 Tbsp tomato paste
2 Tbsp olive oil

Heat 1 Tbsp of olive oil and add sausage to a large pot and cook for approximately 5-8 minutes until cooked through. Removed sausage from pot and set aside. Pour other Tbsp of olive oil into the pot with meat debris and add onion, peppers, and celery into the pot; cook until the onions are translucent. Add some of the salt and pepper to vegetables and cook for approximately 5-8 minutes. Add garlic and continue to cook for approximately 2 more minutes; then add tomato paste and cook for 5-8 minutes or until the mixture is a dark brown, red color.

Add small amount of chicken broth to deglaze the pot and add all seasonings, and the can of roasted diced tomatoes and cook on low/medium heat. Add sausage and chicken into the pot and add additional broth approximately 1/2 cup. Add cauliflower rice to the mixture and combine well; add any additional broth as needed to ensure that the mixture is not dry. (Add the broth slowly to ensure it is also not too soupy) Add parsley to mixture, serve in shallow bowl and enjoy!

Okra Fries

When most think of okra, they envision a stew pot with okra and tomatoes simmering away. However, okra fries have a little bit of a crust with magnificent taste to go along with it. Yes, this is one of our fav's.

Ingredients:

1 lb of cleaned okra
1-2 tsp of salt
1 tsp black pepper
1 tsp granulated garlic
1 Tbsp olive oil

Preheat the oven to 400 degrees F.

In a mixing bowl, place okra, olive oil, and the dry seasonings. Mix thoroughly to ensure that all okra is covered in the mixture. Place in oven and cook for 45 minutes to 1 hour or until the okra has browned slightly and is soft when punctured with fork. These are so great, and you can add grated parmesan or truffle flavored salt to kick it up a notch!

Shepard's Pie with Mashed Cauliflower

Ingredients:

Meat Sauce:

1-lb organic beef and 1-lb organic pork	2 carrots
1 Tbsp minced garlic or 2 fresh cloves minced	1 sm sweet yellow onion
1 Tbsp Tomato paste	1 Tbsp sweet paprika
1/4 cup organic red wine or sherry	1/2 tsp cayenne pepper
1-2 cups of chicken or beef broth	1 tsp oregano
1 small bag of fresh or frozen peas	1 Tbsp granulated garlic
Salt and pepper to taste	

Mashed cauliflower:
1 head organic cauliflower
1/2 cup of unsweetened almond milk, plain
1 stick of organic butter or 1/2 cup ghee
1 tsp granulated garlic
1 cup of Organic white cheddar cheese (omit for clean eating plans)

Steam the cleaned cauliflower head in microwave in a large deep bowl with small amount of water in bottom for approximately 5 minutes or until you are able to easily pierce with fork. In food processer or blender put cauliflower, butter, and granulated garlic; blend, adding the almond milk until a consistency of mashed potatoes is obtained; salt and pepper to taste. Add 1/2 cup of cheese and blend; put the cauliflower aside.

In a large Dutch pot, heat olive oil and add chopped onions and carrots, cooking until soft and translucent; season with salt and pepper. Add garlic and cook additional 5 minutes, stirring to avoid sticking to bottom of pot. Add tomato paste, paprika and granulated garlic and continue to stir for an additional 3-5 minutes, then add sherry to deglaze the pot. Add beef broth and continue to cook on low heat. In a separate frying pan, brown beef and pork and drain thoroughly. Add meat to the sauces and continue to cook for 20 minutes, adding broth as needed. Add the peas to the mixture and stir well; remove from stove and put meat in the bottom of the dish. Cover with mashed cauliflower and top with remaining cheese. Cook at 350 degrees F for approximately 20-25 minutes until cheese is melting and browning and enjoy!

Roasted Broccoli

Ingredients:

2 large broccoli heads or 1 large bag of broccoli florets (hint: go with the bag!)
1 Tbsp of dried Italian seasonings
1-2 tsp of salt
1 tsp black pepper
1/2 tsp red pepper flakes
3 Tbsp ghee or organic butter
1 Tbsp olive oil

Preheat the oven to 400 degrees F.

Place the broccoli florets in a mixing bowl and pour the olive oil and melted butter over the florets; mix thoroughly to ensure that all florets are coated in the oil/butter mixture. Pour the florets into a disposable aluminum pan and generously sprinkle with the seasonings, salt, pepper and pepper flakes. Place in oven and cook for 45 minutes to 1 hour or until the cauliflower has browned slightly and is soft when punctured with fork. This can be topped with a shredded hard cheese or can be accompanied with a feta whipped yogurt cream or just by itself!

Cauliflower Pizza

Ingredients:

1 frozen cauliflower crust
1 cup of leftover Bolognese sauce from last week
1 small pack organic pepperoni slices
1/4 cup of marinated olives, cut in half
1 Tbsp of minced roasted garlic
1 Tbsp dried Italian seasoning
1 large cup of organic mozzarella cheese
1 Tbsp grated asiago cheese
2 basil leaves, chiffon for garnish

Follow instructions on cauliflower crust to preheat oven and prep. On crust, add the Bolognese sauce, spreading evenly with 1/2 inch around the edge of pizza crust. Add the mozzarella cheese, then pepperoni, garlic, and olives to the top. Season with Italian dressing and put in oven directly or on pizza stone; cook per directions on the crust. Remove from oven and sprinkle with the asiago cheese; allow to cool for approximately 5 minutes. Then add the chiffon basil and serve! This is easy. Cut into slices. Recommend 2 slices with a garden salad for lunch or dinner.

Broccoli Muffuletta Salad

New Orleans is known for lots of things, but one is our unique sandwiches called muffulettas. Just a great Italian twist, and we have made this broccoli slaw with that same unique twist. Super easy to make since all the pickled vegetables are in the olive salad, with absolutely tons of flavor! (If you are not a big olive fan, then simply omit the olive salad and follow the dressing idea below)

Ingredients:

1 bag of broccoli slaw (just too easy not to get this; it's one and done!)
1 small jar of Italian olive salad (this is a saltier item, so no added salt to the dish)
1 Tbsp honey
1/2 tsp pepper
2 Tbsp of mozzarella left from the pizza (buffalo balls work great here)
1 Tbsp grated parmesan
2 basil leaves, chiffon for garnish
1 Tbsp slivered almonds for garnish

In a mixing bowl, combine the broccoli slaw with the Italian olive salad and the rest of the ingredients, blending well with tongs. Refrigerate for approximately 1 hour. Garnish with almonds when ready to serve. I seriously can't make a salad any easier than this!

For those who are not big olive fans, simply mix 1 Tbsp balsamic vinegar, 1 Tbsp olive oil, 1 tsp of dried Italian seasonings, 1 tsp minced garlic, 1 tsp honey, salt, and pepper. Whisk well and pour into the broccoli slaw, mixing well with tongs!

PLAY BY PLAY
WEEK SIX
6 Week PREP FOR IT START UP COURSE

The LAST week and you are likely a pro! Congratulations on sticking to the process and developing great habits. Worked through the PEER steps (Prep, Eat, Evaluate, Repeat) to provide you with the greatest chance for success.

Bullet Points:
- The meals that take longer to prepare and cook should be started on first.
- Review the weekly menu and collect all of the ingredients, condiments, and seasonings. Sort with each individual dish/tray.
- Wash all vegetables first to expedite the prep.
- Clean utensils and kitchen equipment as you go to minimize the cleaning in the end.

Supplies:

Parchment Paper	Aluminum Pans (3-4)	Slow cooker
Skillet x 2	Cookie Sheets	Mixing bowls (med, large)
Prep/storage container	Spatula	Tongs x 2
Cutting knives	Cutting board (plastic/wood)	Measuring cups/spoons
Ziplock bags	Whisk or fork	Timer
Vegetable scraper	Dutch oven	Ice cream scoop

- Preheat oven 400 degrees. Sort all the ingredients with the specific recipes, trays or pans.
- Cut vegetables for cacciatore, chop the onions for peppers and pie. Chop carrots, green beans, and de-stem the kale.
- Take clean chicken pieces and season with salt, pepper, and granulated garlic. Dust with almond flour. Braise the chicken in a heated and oiled Dutch oven, when brown place in an aluminum pan. In the existing Dutch oven deglaze the pot, add the onions, tomato paste and sherry, stirring to release the debris on the bottom of the pot. Pour over the chicken. Put the zucchini, squash, olives, onions, and other seasonings according to the recipe to the pan, mix well with tongs. Season again and cover with foil, place in the oven.
- In Dutch oven brown ground meat for peppers and add ingredients according to the recipe stirring often to avoid sticking to the pot. Place the peppers on a plate adding a small amount of water to the plate and microwave for 1-2 minutes until slightly soft and then stuff with the ground meat mixture and top with shredded cheese and put in the oven. Set timer.

WHAT'S EATING YOU?

- Cut the breast, leg and thigh meat off of the rotisserie chicken and cut into cubes. Cut andouille sausage into small cubes. In a large heated skillet add olive oil, and onions cooking until brown, add chicken and sausage cooking until crispy on the edges and continue to follow the recipe adding the cauliflower rice until done. Allow to cool and place in prep or storage containers and then put in the fridge.
- In a large mixing bowl, mix broccoli, olive oil and seasonings with remaining ingredients and mix with tongs. Place ingredients onto 1 half of parchment lined cookie sheet. Same mixing bowl add the green beans with olive oil, seasonings and ingredients put on other side of parchment lined cookie sheet. Then put in the oven.
- Cut spaghetti squash in half, core out seeds with ice cream scoop and brush with olive oil, salt and pepper and place face down in an aluminum pan or parchment lined cookie sheet and set aside.
- In another mixing bowl put kale, olive oil, seasonings together. Mix with tongs and put on 1 half of parchment lined cookie sheet. In the same mixing bowl stir the asparagus, olive oil, seasonings with tongs and put on other half of the parchment lined cookie sheet.
- In a Dutch oven brown ground meat for Shepard's pie adding ingredients per recipe. Can add 1 coup of frozen peas at the end. Make the mashed cauliflower per the recipe with cheese added. In a pie shell or small aluminum pan put the ground meat mixture in the bottom then fold the mashed cauliflower onto the meat mixture and top with cheese. (When cooled put this in the fridge this can be warmed another day as all ingredients are cooked.)
- Remove broccoli and green beans and allow to cool and put in prep or storage containers. Put the spaghetti squash, kale and asparagus into the oven and allow to roast. Uncover the chicken cacciatore at this time.
- Take frozen cauliflower crust out of freezer and add the thawed Bolognese sauce to the crust and then add the remaining pizza ingredients, cheese and olives and set aside.
- Remove the kale and asparagus allow them to cool and put the pizza in the oven and set the timer. When chicken pulling from bone remove the chicken cacciatore and allow to cool.
- Remove the spaghetti squash when soft and can be punctured with fork, allowing to cool. Once cool can shred with a fork and then add the sauce and chicken from catchettorie and put in prep or storage container. Pick up all disposable equipment/utensils and wash remaining dishes and bowls.

Snack-N-Go

When working through the first 6 weeks of the starter program, I usually recommend abstaining from any snacking and if needed, eat 5 smaller meals instead of the traditional 3 meals that we have been accustomed. However, if you feel that a snack between the 3 smaller meals of the day would bode well for you, we have provided a list of options that could effectively manage those "hangry" pangs that we know all too well. Your snack, if you choose to partake in one should be lower in calorie, low carbohydrate, with as many organic ingredients as possible. Remember, portion control is the thing. Just because it is healthy or packed with protein doesn't mean that it is low in calories. Always keep in mind, a calorie is a calorie is a calorie!

- Nuts, dry roasted preferred. (However, if possible, avoid peanuts, they are not technically a nut.) Many nuts come shelled and ready to go, making this a very mobile snack.
- Red and Yellow Bell pepper slices with guacamole.
- Apple slices with almond butter
- Celery sticks with pimento cheese
- Kale chips (this isn't just for a side dish!) see our recipe in the 6-week course.
- Beef jerky (there are many great brands, organic no sugar rec.)
- Whey Protein bars/shakes
- Almond or coconut milk protein yogurt with berries
- Skinny almonds
- Cucumber slices with hummus
- Cauliflower pretzels with soft cheese
- Parmesan cheese crisps (can easily be made at home)
- String cheese

- Heirloom tomatoes with Mozzarella Cheese
- Boiled Eggs
- Baby Carrots with Blue Cheese or Ranch Dressing
- Dried Fruit (Be careful to watch the carbohydrates with this option)
- Turkey Roll-up with almond milk cream cheese.
- Marinated Olives
- Avocado with buffalo sauce

COVID, Corona... Tomato, Tumato
Afterthoughts

As I began the arduous task of putting the initial editing changes into the book, I personally, as well as those around me, began to experience an unprecedented pandemic. COVID-19 monopolized conversations, affected our "business as usual," and became a catalyst for many emotional eaters. Life as we knew it has and still is drastically changing. For many, they were left to work within the confines of their homes or even worse, left unemployed, lacking the necessary resources to provide for their healthy lifestyle. During the lock-downs, as an essential worker, I still provided care for emergency visits and obstetrical patients. However, even my role and schedule had been drastically affected. The emotions during traumatic times have been running very high, leaving many with the temptation to let the emotional monster out of the cage to stretch his legs a bit. I implore you to really concentrate and focus on the end goal during this time, and make sure that extra efforts are being implemented to thwart off the temptations of comfort eating.

    As this "new normal" has settled in, many patients have come in for their routine visits, and frequently the first comment I hear upon entering the exam room is, "I have gained so much weight!" Instead of dealing with the "Freshman 15," a term used by many to account for the unexplained 15-pound weight gain that occurs for many college freshman. My patients were wrestling with "COVID 19." We laugh a little about the changes in our lifestyle during these visits, but many have succumbed to the emotional monster's diabolical tactics to wreak havoc to our overall wellness and health. Whether they are eating more comfort foods, having more evening cocktails, or have reincorporated an evening dessert into the mix, the results are inevitably the same.

So, Kelly, what do I do? These are truly unprecedented times, so how do you "prepare" for something like this? Gheez, these are really good questions. I don't know if there is one specific way that you can truly be completely prepared for this type of event. However, to avoid the downward spiral of binge, or comfort eating, it is more important than ever to ensure your PREP FOR IT steps are being fully utilized and constantly evaluated. When we realized that we would be in a "lockdown" mode for a few weeks and might not be able to frequent the grocery stores, like many, we started stocking up on the essentials (Not just toilet paper!). Something that I noticed as we were loading our inventory into the grocery cart, is many of the healthy options, almond flour, coconut oil, etc. were still very accessible. Many shelves that housed cookies, cakes, chips, and bread were left barren. However, the foods that are most beneficial to an emotional eater, were left untouched. It is in these troubled times, that we must be incredibly focused on the goal, identifying the potential pitfalls, and create healthy alternative options to stay the course. The PREP FOR IT steps were developed to prompt you to ask the hard questions during the difficult times. This would include a global pandemic!

My husband is a safe driving instructor for his company and has to certify many of the engineers who are driving company vehicles. Much like our PREP FOR IT steps, the company used the Smiths System to provide the drivers with quick, useful phrases to reinforce good driving behaviors. One phrase, used by the drivers to prevent collisions and drive safer is, "All Good Kids Love Milk." What? That doesn't make a lick of sense, Kelly! You're right, it doesn't. But each word in the phrase prompts the driver to remember certain measures to provide proactively during their daily driving schedules.

- The first word, "All" represented "Aim high in steering." Simply put, when you are making your way through the busy highways, keep your focus or gaze high and looking

ahead for potential issues. For you, it's imperative that you are aiming high and anticipating some pitfalls with food accessibility and meal choices.
- The second word, stands for "get the big picture." Make sure that you have scoped out your entire surroundings and identified culprits. Make sure that your pantry, desk drawer, and even your car, are void of any food temptations.
- "Keep your eyes moving" refers to being alert and aware of the surroundings as you are driving. In our PREP FOR IT steps, this could prompt you to be aware of situations or issues that could elicit emotional triggers. Occasionally, stop yourself for a moment and assess your situation in your mind, working through the potential issues you may have identified. Reduce emotional highs and lows that could result in unwanted, reactive choices. Keep your eyes peeled for situations and issues that could offset your goal of overall wellness and health.
- "Like" represents, leave yourself an out. In other words, when the potential for a reactive choice is more likely, then provide a window of escape to ensure you stay the course. Have an alternative plan in place for a meal or snack if the initial plan doesn't pan out. In addition, you may have found yourself looking for alternatives to your weekly workouts with many gym closures. As we started getting information about the potential lockdowns, I started researching apps and programs that I could use to work out within the confines of our 4 walls. I realized my normal routine would be affected and a plan needed to be implemented BEFORE it was needed to ensure a smooth transition.
- Finally, the last word stands for "Make sure they see you." To avoid a collision while driving, you may hit the horn (my husband often thinks I overuse this car accessory!) to ensure the unaware driver is alerted to your presence. In relation to our PREP FOR IT STEPS, it's imperative to recognize the potential emotional issues and even

call them out to prevent a reactive response. As silly as this may sound, calling the emotion out will allow you to take the measures necessary ahead of time to prevent crashes when the time comes. Sometimes utilizing the accountability partner we mentioned earlier to assist you with likely pitfalls and discussing some alternative measures and what the "out" may look like, can be most beneficial. Your most effective weapon against the emotional monster's dubious ploy to throw you off course is to call the emotional monster out and tell him to pack his bags; he isn't welcome here!

Whether you are dealing with a stressful day at work, a death of a loved one, or even a pandemic of unfathomable proportions, follow your PREP FOR IT steps. Make them part of your daily routine like brushing your teeth or drinking that first cup of coffee before the workday begins. Wear out the tools and resources that have been provided to you. Doing this will not only allow you to achieve your health and wellness goals, but will also place the emotional monster into permanent confinement!

We would love to continue to be there for you during your wellness and weight loss journey. Stay up-to-date, with the prep4it.com website for additional recipes, prep-rallies, new tips and product reviews.

References and Background Reading

The Honeymooners Quotes. https://screenrant.com/honeymooners-ralph-gleason-quotes-hilarious-today/

Klok MD, Jakobsdottir S, Drent ML. "The role of leptin and ghrelin in the regulation of food intake and body weight in humans: a review." Obes Rev. 2007 Jan;8(1):21-34. doi: 10.1111/j.1467-789X.2006.00270.x.

Ghrelin: The "Hunger Hormone" Explained. https://www.healthline.com/nutrition/ghrelin

Feedback Loop Images. https://www.gameofficials.com/queensland/video-feedback-loop-tutorial.php

Pearls before breakfast: Can One of the Nation's Greatest Musicians Cut through the Fog of a D.C. Rush Hour? Let's Find out. https://www.washingtonpost.com/lifestyle/magazine/pearls-before-breakfast-can-one-of-the-nations-great-musicians-cut-through-the-fog-of-a-dc-rush-hour-lets-find-out/2014/09/23/8a6d46da-4331-11e4-b47c-f5889e061e5f_story.html

Body Shapes Image. https://www.shutterstock.com/image-vector/vector-illustrations-collection-multiethnic-characters-body-positive-1719324640

Aesop's Fables for Children: The Fox and the Grapes. http://read.gov/aesop/005.html

How to Overcome 5 Psychological Blocks to Weight Loss. Frey, M. https://www.verywellfit.com/overcome-emotional-stress-to-lose-weight-3495947

Clear, J. "Atomic Habits". New York City: Random House, 2018; pages 13-16.

13 Steps to Stop Making Excuses and Get Results in Your Life. https://www.developgoodhabits.com/making-excuses/

Adages on Hard Work. https://www.goodreads.com/quotes/24889-the-three-great-essentials-to-achieve-anything-worthwhile-are first#:~:text=Quote%20by%20Thomas%20A.%20Edison%3A%20%E2%80%9CThe%20three%20great,friends%20thought%20of%20this%20quote%2C%20please%20sign%20up%21

https://www.quoteambition.com/calvin-coolidge-quotes/#:~:text=Calvin%20Coolidge%20Quotes%20on%20Hard%20Work%20and%20Business,or%20intellectually%2C%20without%20effort%3B%20and%20effort%20means%20work.%E2%80%9D

SMART Goals. https://goalsetting.org/smart-goals

Steps to Prep, Red Cross. https://www.redcross.org/get-help/how-to-prepare-for-emergencies.html

Hanbury, S. "How to Emotionally Prepare for a Hurricane" https://www.apa.org/topics/disasters-response/hurricane-preparation

Paleo. Dr Loren Cordain https://thepaleodiet.com/author/loren

WW. copyright. https://www.weightwatchers.com/us

BMI Harris Benedict Equation BMI app https://www.bmi-calculator.net/bmr-calculator/harris-benedict-equation

https://bmicalc.org/resources/harris-benedict-equation

https://www.cdc.gov/healthyweight/assessing/bmi/adult_bmi/english_bmi_calculator/bmi_calculator.html

USDH 5 Major Food Groups. https://www.usda.gov/media/blog/2017/09/26/back-basics-all-about-myplate-food-groups

GMO definition. https://en.wikipedia.org/wiki/Genetically_modified_organism

Allocations for metabolism https://www.mayoclinic.org/healthy-lifestyle/weight-loss/in-depth/metabolism

National Center for Health Statistics Rate of Obesity https://www.cdc.gov/nchs/data/databriefs/db288.pdf

Hart, C. Grossman, M.K. "The Insulin Resistance Diet". 2 Pennsylvania Plaza, New York City: McGraw-Hill Education; 2nd edition, 2007; pages 35-58.

The Story of Charlie Brown. https://en.wikipedia.org/wiki/Charlie_Brown

National Alliance on Mental Illness Stats. https://www.nimh.nih.gov/health/statistics/mental-illness

Obesity Action Coalition. https://www.obesityaction.org/

Winch, G. "Seven Habits of Highly Emotional Healthy Individuals" Psychology Today. https://www.psychologytoday.com/intl/blog/the-squeaky-wheel/201307/the-7-habits-highly-emotionally-healthy-people

Tracy, B. "Eat That Frog! 21 Great Ways to Stop Procrastinating and Get More Done in Less Time". San Francisco: Berret-Koehler Publishers, Inc. 2009; pages 1-6.

5 Rules of the Smith System https://www.topdriver.com/education-blog/5-rules-of-the-smith-system/

Made in the USA
Coppell, TX
17 May 2023

16940997R10152